Health Research in Practice

Volume Two
Personal experiences, public issues

Edited by

Derek Colquhoun

*Faculty of Education, Deakin University,
Geelong, Australia*

and

Allan Kellehear

*School of Sociology and Anthropology, La Trobe University,
Melbourne, Australia*

CHAPMAN & HALL

London · Glasgow · Weinheim · New York · Tokyo · Melbourne · Madras

Published by Chapman & Hall, 2–6 Boundary Row, London SE1 8HN, UK

Chapman & Hall, 2–6 Boundary Row, London SE1 8HN, UK

Blackie Academic & Professional, Wester Cleddens Road, Bishopbriggs, Glasgow G64 2NZ, UK

Chapman & Hall GmbH, Pappelallee 3, 69469 Weinheim, Germany

Chapman & Hall USA, 115 Fifth Avenue, New York NY 10003, USA

Chapman & Hall Japan, ITP-Japan, Kyowa Building, 3F, 2-2-1 Hirakawacho, Chiyoda-ku, Tokyo 102, Japan

Chapman & Hall Australia, 102 Dodds Street, South Melbourne, Victoria 3205, Australia

Chapman & Hall India, R. Seshadri, 32 Second Main Road, CIT East, Madras 600 035, India

Distributed in the USA and Canada by Singular Publishing Group Inc., 4284 41st Street, San Diego, California 92105

First edition 1996

© 1996 Chapman & Hall

Typeset in 10/12pt Palatino by Saxon Graphics Ltd, Derby

Printed in England by Clays Ltd., St Ives plc

ISBN 0 412 62330 7   1 56593 608 6   (USA)

A catalogue record for this book is available from the British Library

Library of Congress Catalog Card Number: 95-74651

∞ Printed on permanent acid-free text paper, manufactured in accordance with ANSI/NISO Z39.48-1992 and ANSI/NISO Z39.48-1984 (Permanence of Paper).

For Sue, Ewan, Callum and Rowan

Contents

Contributors

Frances Baum Associate Professor of Community Medicine, Flinders University of South Australia, Adelaide, Australia

Derek Colquhoun Senior Lecturer in Health Education, Deakin University, Geelong, Australia

Pat Crotty Senior Lecturer in Nutrition Education, Deakin University, Geelong, Australia

David Field Professor of Sociology, University of Ulster, Jordanstown, Northern Ireland, UK

Margaret Hamilton Associate Professor of Drug and Alcohol Studies, University of Melbourne, Australia

Lyn Harrison Postgraduate in Education, Deakin University, Geelong, Australia

Allan Kellehear Senior Lecturer in Sociology, La Trobe University, Melbourne, Australia

Glenda Koutroulis Postgraduate in Sociology, La Trobe University, Melbourne, Australia

Karen Lane Associate Lecturer in Sociology, Deakin University, Geelong, Australia

Beverley Raphael Professor of Psychiatry, University of Queensland, Brisbane, Australia

Pranee Liamputtong Rice Senior Lecturer in Sociology, La Trobe University, Melbourne, Australia

Gwenneth Roberts Senior Research Officer, Department of Psychiatry, University of Queensland, Brisbane, Australia

David Stephens Research Officer, National Centre for HIV Social Research, Melbourne, Australia

Preface

The first volume of *Health Research in Practice* was underpinned by the belief that abstract, theoretical and methodological discussions of health research failed to grasp the deeper, broader complexities that characterize this area. Research is always conducted by men and women who are confronted by an assortment of political, ethical and methodological pressures, which are seldom discussed in the more theoretical treatments of health research. This is because personal experience is so often sanitized, even erased, from so many textbook accounts of research practice.

Sometimes the pressures to which researchers are subject threaten their very research aims or conclusions. Sometimes such pressures may radically modify our attitude or conduct toward those we research, or toward those who fund or employ us. At other times, health research in practice critically revises our understanding of fundamental taken-for-granted ideas such as 'politics', 'ethics', 'representation' or 'theory'.

The purpose of this second volume, then, is to continue and extend our exploration of these issues. It represents our ongoing belief that critical reflections on actual research practice are our best defence against ethically irresponsible, politically naive research practices. Only if students and practitioners of health research are exposed to a broad and diverse range of personal experiences which shape the practical conduct of health research, will we be better prepared to meet those challenges.

The first volume presented twelve voices, twelve experiences of health research in practice. In this second volume we present the reader with another twelve experiences which test and reflect the ethical and political tensions in health research. Most of the early chapters examine personal experiences of confronting the unpredictable politics of university life, competitive grant applications or simply attempting to represent and study 'the other'.

However, just as we did in the first volume, we also present the reader with some reflections on the gap between the theory and practice of certain methods used in health research. In Volume one we discussed the phenomenological method, the survey and the historical approach to health research. In this volume we discuss the techniques of memory work, the study of existing sources and the use of interviewing.

Finally, this volume ends with three discussions about the broader political influences on health research today. These chapters are devoted to a discussion of the important, ongoing problem of the medicalization of health. The tendency for positivist biomedical ideas to capture and dominate health ideas in the areas of childbirth, nutrition and health promotion is taken up in those final chapters. In these ways the current volume continues to address the two most important pressures that confront every health researcher: the abstract public issues and personal experience of these in the everyday, face-to-face world of health research in practice.

Margaret Hamilton begins the book with a poignant account of 'the vicissitudes' of running a research team when most of that team are funded by short-term research monies. Her research team works in drugs and alcohol, an area that easily attracts funding and public attention, but both universities and the wider community display much ambivalence towards it, which often translates, in practical terms, into short-term, unreliable funding and unwanted public attention.

Derek Colquhoun continues to look at the politics of funding but extends his discussion to focus on the biomedical bias which places limits on qualitative research projects. He takes us on a short tour of his experiences and research projects and suggests alternative ways of researching the area.

Pranee Liamputtong Rice begins a set of three chapters which looks at the problem of representation. Rice argues that all research depends on the good faith and cooperation of those we wish to study, but for those from a non-English-speaking background cooperation with researchers has its perils. Rice attempts to extrapolate from her experience with such people some principles which may help others avoid some of the social and ethical pitfalls.

David Stephens has quite a different problem: he reflects on the dilemmas of studying a group of which he is a member. In this case, Stephens examines and reflects on the strengths and weaknesses of studying those who are HIV positive when the researcher is also HIV positive. However, the situation is somewhat complicated by the fact that having the same virus does not necessarily mean automatic or total identification. This is because identification has much to do with a shared mode of transmission – something David did not have.

Lyn Harrison takes this issue further by posing the question of representation afresh. How is it possible to represent 'the other'? Harrison chronicles her attempt to employ empowering methods in her study of young women, but then identifies the problems of those assumptions in practice. She cautions against an instrumentalist view of methods and politics, arguing that both validity and empowerment are themselves discursive practices. The problems of representation cannot be overcome simply by good intentions. Harrison argues that we need to overturn simple, mechanistic notions of power to see that, although inevitably heirarchical, its effects are multiple and not always repressive.

Glenda Koutroulis' chapter is the first of three whose focus is specifically on method. Koutroulis describes her use of memory work with a group of women recalling their first menstrual experience. She discusses the theory of the method as proposed in various research articles, and then reflects on the problems she encountered in the execution of the method in her study.

Kellehear asks, where has all the methodological diversity gone in health research? He quickly reviews the basis for his belief that the interview and survey dominate health research before using his study of the near-death experience as an example of how other methods can be equally or more fruitful to health researchers. The focus of his attention is the use of existing sources.

Field returns our gaze to the interview once more, and describes his 'road test' of this method in nursing research. His basic problem was, as he describes it, being the inexpert expert. How does a non-health professional, indeed a non-nurse, conduct research into nursing work? He chronicles the problems and the wisdom of hindsight in his research with those nursing the dying.

Raphael and Roberts continue this interest in the nurse–researcher by examining the political and ethical issues of research in accident and emergency settings. The role of the nurse–researcher is one that has distinct advantages and disadvantages at different times. The developmental process and the political negotiations behind such research are described and some lessons drawn for the unwary.

Finally, Lane, Crotty and Baum discuss the general problem of medicalization in three different guises. Lane argues that medical authorities have colonized the debate over birthing options and discusses the methodological implications of this for research in Australia and the UK. Crotty examines the problem of the assumption in much nutrition research that the only worthwhile questions to ask are ones that might lead to dietary improvement, but is this true? If not, what are the methodological implications of this answer?

Baum examines the way public health has changed over the past two decades and is now settling around the issue of health promotion. She discusses the demands of research work in community settings and argues the need for diverse methodologies. Drawing from her experience with the Healthy Cities project she illustrates some of the possibilities here. And although there are still constant pressures to promote more research into weight loss or smoking cessation, Baum argues that research into these communities show health researchers the need to:

> .....be more inventive with the techniques they use, communicate effectively to develop partnerships with community practitioners and the communities they work with and keep their theoretical heads above the hubble and bubble of community action to see how the particular case fits more general knowledge and theory.

These words summarize our hopes and aims for *Health Research in Practice Volume Two*. Good reading!

Derek Colquhoun and Allan Kellehear

CHAPTER 1

The vicissitudes of running a research team

Margaret Hamilton

I never imagined I would do research. I went to university in order to acquire the necessary qualifications to do the sort of work I wanted to do, which at that time was social work. From a childhood in rural Australia I had been shocked into political consciousness by a year of living in the Philippines, and returned to Australia young, energized and naively politicized. I am no longer young; I sometimes long for energy and come dangerously close to resigned cynicism. Still, I retain curiosity, determination and a concern for justice which impels me and lies behind my struggles to maintain a research team.

This chapter will examine the issues associated with directing a research team where funding is soft, ethics are ambiguous, the host organization is ambivalent and the environment is unquiet and controversial, with multiple audiences. The team must respond to interests ranging from policy makers, programme planners and clinical practitioners to politicolegal interests and users of various substances. Most areas are contested and, while the area of interest is topical today, its future is uncertain. Maintaining a research team in the drug and alcohol field can be both seductive and offputting. This is an environment where young researchers from a range of disciplines gather, intrigued and committed to exploration and mixed methodologies, and where most are on appointments of less than 6 months.

THE RESEARCH AGENDA

The Drug and Alcohol Research Team or Teaching Unit (DART) is a multidisciplinary group with a history of involvement with applied issues in the context of research in the alcohol and drug area. The special expertise of our group centres particularly on the social aspects of drug and alcohol research. A commitment to links with the practice and policy world arises in an understanding that people in the alcohol and drug world, like others, are confronted with growing demands for relevance and accountability; an exponential growth in relevant research and literature; increasing demands for programme management and quality assurance ; an increase in the diversity of expertise required to understand and manage alcohol and drug problems, and shrinking resources for addressing these demands on a programme-by-programme basis.

The research agenda has evolved rather than arising from some carefully planned strategy or adoption of a mission statement. We did articulate general guiding principles early in our development and we have attempted to maintain them; we know what we are not likely to do rather than the areas that we are likely to pursue. We have found it difficult to be proactive in setting a more definitive research agenda as it is dependent on the personnel and the availability of funding, and thus largely other people's priorities.

DART research includes applied, action and evaluation research as well as exploratory/descriptive work, some of which might reasonably be regarded as theoretical research. Arising from my own interest and that of some of the team we have a particular focus on women and alcohol, but might also be identified in researching hidden drug-using populations. The little-respected area of evaluation research is where we have been most successful in acquiring funds.

Our project funding ranges from nil (for the many one-off consultations to community groups and small programmes) to a project over 3 years totalling some $250,000. We have taken our evaluation research projects well beyond pragmatic questioning and it is here that some of the most lively debates about epistemology, relevance and utility and mixed methods take place.

The culture that has emerged within the research group has allowed stimulus, sufficient mentorship and diversity to retain staff and attract higher degree students. Its future at this time is most uncertain, and the story that follows is one which deliberately contains elements of both personal or private troubles and public or research issues.

The research team was not created because of someone's felt need or as a result of a specific grant. It arose from my interest and initial success in gaining funding at a time when drug and alcohol concerns were a 'flavour of the year' which, although gradually diminishing, has lasted for some 8 years. It has had rapid growth, which is both its strength and its weakness, and now includes 11 core members (whose work is predominantly DART work) and seven others (including part-time higher degree students) as well as other associates.

DART now comprises:

- one full-time research fellow (foundation discipline in psychology);
- two full-time research assistants (psychology, sociology);

- three research fellows/assistants who are at least half time (social sciences, policy studies, social work);
- three other research assistants who are less than half time (medicine, statistics, social work);
- one occasional project worker (social sciences).

It also includes scholarship and fellowship holders:

- one full-time post-doctoral fellow (pharmacology);
- three full-time PhD students (anthropology, sociology/psychology, educational psychology);
- one research Master's student (psychology/sociology/women's studies);
- three other part-time PhD students (medicine, nursing, social work).

There are other casual workers, including occasional interviewers and a graphic artist assisting with a computer-assisted learning-related educational research project. Two full-time associates are located elsewhere (with backgrounds in psychology and human nutrition). Other professional associates include medical practitioners, nurse practitioners and criminologists.

FROM PRACTICE TO RESEARCH

No-one in an academic environment over the past 20 years can fail to have noticed that one ultimately stands or falls on research activity. Notwithstanding the considerable rhetoric about the importance of teaching, discussion with anyone who has served on promotion and selection committees in most tertiary education institutions reveals the importance of research.

In my early days in academia my effort, like so many of my professional colleagues', went to teaching; to the responsibility for the next generation of my own profession; to the individuals, families, groups and organizations that these graduates would work with; to their acquisition of fundamental knowledge, skills and professional culture, and to a preoccupation with practice competence. There was little time for research and little respect for it among those who had come 'from practice'. Those of us who were practitioners saw our credibility and authority arising in the real world – the world separate from ivory towers, the world of practice wisdom and 'doing'. Research seemed quite different and remote.

I came to research through practice. I had done research courses and research projects as a graduate student and had used research to examine supervision and skills transmission in the professional curriculum. While being centrally involved in teaching social work, I maintained an ongoing interest in the drug and alcohol field which had been an area of my direct practice. It was never static and involved a range of disciplines. It was a field rich in ideas and opportunities; it could, for example, span the study of literature through the biographies of famous drug users and drunkards; the intricacies of neurotransmitters and the chemistry of the brain; the moral and legal complexities of proscribing human behaviours; agricultural policies in developing nations and the international marketing of drugs, and an array of applied knowledge from public health to economics and law enforcement.

My formal career as a researcher began on an almost casual basis. Sending a letter asking to be kept in touch with whoever responded to a general flyer about work that was needed in a remote Australian mining town where alcohol had been identified as a problem, I found myself being invited to do the research. A modest budget allowed for the employment of a research assistant and some travel money. Very soon I was plunged into a world of considerable practical and political complexity. This meant much learning on the job; consulting as we went along; developing methods to suit the environment; working with the critical audiences to the research, and straddling the complex political web of a company town. It was here that my first efforts in gaining access – examining the available research tools, testing them for applicability in this environment and talking to people – really started.

Of course, not everything in life, not even research, exists in an emotional and social vacuum. For me this first struggle to master larger-scale research was profoundly affected by the momentous upheaval of my personal life as I became pregnant for the first time, gave birth to a son and endured his subsequent illness and death at 7 months of age.

The next milestone in my career occurred as a result of my field of interest receiving a significant boost in funding through the launch, in 1986, of the National Campaign Against Drug Abuse (NCADA). This initiative emerged from a landscape of unanticipated Prime Ministerial tears on national television and rising concern about drug abuse in the community. Fortunately, the Australian effort was hijacked early in its development and emerged to include a focus on licit as well as illicit drugs.

The alcohol and drug field went from being an eccentric fascination to a vehicle for resource expenditure, seeking theoretical and other inputs from many disciplines. It was in this environment that my shift from social work occurred. Owing more to serendipity than sound strategic planning, I was keen to try to assist those programmes who were seeking and, in many cases, receiving money to respond to the item in funding applications which asks 'How do you propose to evaluate your programme?'

A research proposal to work with a group of programmes to develop some self-evaluation models and tools arose. When this was funded, and I was able to appoint a research assistant for 3 years, my identity as a researcher was public. During this time I was invited on to an evaluation task force to evaluate the first 3 years of the NCADA, projecting my newly acquired status nationally and providing me with further on-the-job learning to add to my already expanded repertoire of skills.

FROM FOUNDATION DISCIPLINE TO HEALTH

One of the initiatives of the second phase of development of the national effort in this field was to allocate funds to all medical schools in the country to employ half-time coordinators of alcohol and drug education. Based on a similar programme in the USA, the belief was that if the quality of service to the general population with alcohol and drug problems was to change significantly, it was necessary to influence the teaching of one of the primary service professions – medicine. 'What better way to provide this influence than to purchase it and implant it in the undergraduate teaching programme of all medical students?' These positions were advertised in the respective medical schools, one in my own university.

I thought it likely that only a medical graduate would be acceptable. I did, however, have a range of experience, including clinical practice, teaching, training, some completed research and, importantly, a research grant. I was selected for the job and told there had been a number of 'suitably qualified medical practitioner' applicants.

RESEARCH: A STRATEGIC INITIATIVE

Although the effort to develop an appropriate curriculum for this audience was challenging, the more difficult task was gaining access to the already crowded timetable. However, through a mix of deliberate planning, taking opportunities that arose and a willingness to contribute in other areas, I was able to develop new inputs on alcohol and drugs and establish professional and practice credibility for my topic. I knew from experience that for this to endure, research credibility was essential. Having worked in a large hospital I also knew that authority with medical students and graduates rested with doctors. The rest of us will only ever achieve associate status: we are visitors, greeted politely and given opportunities, but, ultimately, visitors none the less.

I thus moved to identify medical colleagues whom I could encourage as collaborators and to build a research presence that could provide legitimacy for the curriculum I was delivering. The latter would be critical for any chance to be retained in the faculty when the specific grant ended.

After this initial 3 years, the Faculty negotiated with the State Health Department to have my own salary covered for a further 5 years. While this was not ideal, involving as it did a commitment to providing advice, consultation and input into government services (with them assuming my almost full availability), it did mean that the research team could continue and had an ongoing home.

THE MULTIDISCIPLINARY TEAM

This overused descriptive term turns even its most avid admirers off. It has become a platitude in most worlds and has lost much of its usefulness as a concept. It does, however, describe DART.

Multidisciplinary: why and what does in mean?

The very nature of alcohol- and drug-related research propels us to engage with a range of disciplines and interests. The study of human beings using substances to achieve change in complex social environments with potentially harmful consequences is, by necessity, an endeavour which calls on a range of knowledge. The DART mix is not accidental. When recruiting staff, we consider primarily the needs of the specific project and then the contribution that this person might make to the team.

Multidisciplinary means more than putting people from different disciplines together. Just as triangulation of research approaches can produce more than the sum of the parts, so too does a mix of disciplines. It allows freedom to think and challenge in ways that seem liberating compared to my experience of same-discipline environments.

Having more than one representative of any discipline is better than solo representatives. This helps to identify that which is discipline specific and separates it from personal or subspecialty differences; it facilitates discourse (since the individuals can debate within and between disciplines); and it provides a peer reference group for the purposes of supervision and discipline-specific review. This is critical in an area with a short and somewhat circumscribed career path. Team members need to maintain contact with their foundation disciplines. The drug and alcohol area needs people who update themselves and are stimulated and nurtured by the developments in their foundation fields, since much of the knowledge is derivative.

The dangers inherent in enclaving ourselves in a world of drug and alcohol researchers and workers can be self-destructive. An example of this is the research that proceeded for many years on alcohol and the family. With careful observational studies, attempts at theoretical conceptualization produced some limited typologies, including titles such as 'Whining Winnie', 'Suffering Susan', and 'Controlling Catherine' (Whalen, 1953). Others tried to identify sequential phases of family breakdown within the 'alcoholic family' (Jackson, 1954). It was not until a social psychologist examined these developments in the context of the literature on families with troubles (from variable aetiologies) that the parallels were drawn. These 'alcoholic families' broadly resembled other families that were in 'trouble' where there was no alcohol consumption at all (Orford, 1975).

Cultural differences

Working with different disciplines requires the development of mutual respect, a common language and the ability to give one another due recognition. Perhaps even harder is the importance of having sufficient confidence and trust to offer criticism, or at least question and challenge ideas that arise in a 'foreign' tradition. This makes for considerable debate and turmoil. It is also what provides the creative energy in the team and represents the origins of some of our most difficult but important lessons.

For example, in the process of reviewing the interviews being conducted by two researchers on an evaluation project examining the outcomes of treatment in a therapeutic community, tension arose when it was apparent that one almost always completed all questionnaire items and the other often had incomplete sections. The relationship between the two researchers had been very positive in the preceding months. Part of the study included follow-up interviews with previous clients and used a quasi-experimental design. In trying to understand this world, it followed key informant consultations, focus group discussions, a shared 3-day-and-night residential stay in the community for the researchers with the client/subject group, and observation.

In exploring the differences in data completion, the following explanation arose: the one with completed questionnaires came from a behavioural psychology background. He had been trained to do this, recognizing the problems caused by missing data in quantitative analysis. The other researcher was a social worker and said he thought it improper to record information that was either 'forced' from the subject or invalid. He said it did not make sense to record responses that had no meaning and were offered in a manner which suggested they were either flippant or without substance. He also said that he sometimes chose not to ask some of the more sensitive questions if, in his judgement, it meant that the subject would be significantly upset or unlikely to continue the interview. Both had a legitimate point and their responses were firmly consistent with their foundation disciplines' codes of conduct. Together they represent both the science and the art of the interview. The ensuing debate produced a shift from both and much more meaningful responses. This also shows the subtle differences in professional codes of ethics which emerge in our team, arising from discipline socialization differences.

Distinct disciplines bring myriad subtle differences as well as alternative bodies of knowledge. They might usefully be thought of as families or tribes, each contributing its own cultural traditions, language, practices and ways of communicating. The differences in the discourse of anthropologists and behavioural psychologists, for example, challenge all that is said above about mutual respect for different traditions! While one group seeks for the meaning of their own lived experiences and those of others, the other seeks to partialize, dissect and measure in a manner they describe as objective. The fundamental differences in these exchanges at times require translation. Over time, however, I have seen a transformation and a growth in respect that some might be surprised by.

The nature of the published work in disciplines reveals a difference not only in style but also in quantity. I observe anthropologists as being less driven to produce than the behavioural psychologists. One view might be to consider what is valued by each group. Medical members and others from the more applied professions (such as nursing and social work) are pragmatists. They are keen to know about the applications of new knowledge and to explore ways of using information. They can be captured to reflect and some see value in so doing. Their 'real world' orientation is dominant and can at times be limiting.

At the same time, the theoretical reveries of some of the more theoretically oriented can also be limiting. It seems clear that in a health environment, failure to attend to questions of applicability and utility in research can leave the researchers vulnerable.

Maximizing the mix(?)

Our way of dealing with these tensions is to do a mix of research and garner a range of opportunities from most projects. This allows for some projects to be closer to theorizing and reflection and others to assume the methods or models that concentrate on applications and evaluations of effectiveness. In our team this is an artificial distinction, where apparently contradictory research approaches coexist in parallel studies of the same phenomenon. For example, a significant current project for the team is a study of self-help groups, with one sub-study pursuing the measurement of spirituality through the development and validation of an appropriate set of questions/instruments and another DART member exploring the meaning of the self-help experience, with observation, talking, listening and thinking, i.e. 'being there'.

While the mix of cultures now current in DART makes for a richer research environment, it can also represent the seeds of inefficiency and mismanagement in the current environment, where goals and targets are measured by concrete outputs and resources are stretched. One of our current projects, located in a rural community, has involved a number of DART staff and included epidemiological work seeking evidence to explore a local concern about illicit drug use mixed with consultation with local gatekeepers; observations in local hotels of serving and drinking practices in an attempt to make meaning of the culture; conversations with older people about their use of medications and their stories of a flood within the year which represents loss and grief; the reading of newspaper articles and using these data; the poring over large, leatherbound ledgers at the local police station while noting the language and practices of the police as they go about their work, and reflecting on the meaning of words such as 'tidy', 'clean', and 'neat', which permeate some focus group interviews.

The explicit output of this project will be the report to the auspicing body, the local government council. Implicit gains can enrich the research team. However, it is this balancing of the explicit demands and internal needs that stretches project resources. The fascination with the subject can produce a lack of focus and closure can be difficult. We know that the programme we have evaluated is really wanting the good news story and projects such as this are always time limited. The active players in the project have limited use of any substantial report; they will no longer be employed. The intrinsic value of doing the research must be more than this final, negotiated report, but if we properly costed our effort it would be significantly more than we have been paid.

TEAMS

The formal title of DART does not include the term 'team'. This was its origin but on the advice of more senior members of our faculty we changed the T to represent Teaching Unit. While this was constructed as a management device (the division of the areas of activity of the department being conceptualized and called units), it also represents a reflection on the sense that 'teams' are soft, seventies style, inefficient and old hat in the health arena.

There are set shared roles in which all DART members participate, such as rostered minute taking and mail opening, and individual members sometimes represent DART on outside bodies. There are other informal occasions from time to time which include all or most members, with no one person systematically absent, such as annual, residential long weekends akin to a retreat, where a mix of work and pleasure provides an alternative venue for team reflection and planning.

Teams as research and management structures

The size of the overall unit is a factor in team functioning. When this group comprised four or five members there was a strong sense of cohesion, but it also made for conformity. As the group has expanded subgroups have formed and sometimes these might be described as temporary splits, although their internal composition sometimes alters. It nevertheless remains a cohesive whole.

Most of the projects within DART are also run by sub-groups or teams. Some tension emerges in doing this. Finding a balance between independence and interdependence differs for individuals and projects. Getting the balance right does not always come easily. When staff are paired on a project and start work with DART at the same time, there is a tendency for considerable mutual reliance in the early phase. Discovering their unique contributions can take some time.

The question of who to include and how many to involve in any one project arises from time to time. With such a rich pool to draw on, it is tempting to have a variety of inputs on many projects. It seems important to limit this, however, except for quite specific purposes. We try to allow seminars as an opportunity for tapping the ideas of other team members but occasionally there might be a specific reason for including a range of perspectives.

One such example comes from our study of the curative elements of self-help groups. Here we were keen to enter the world of these groups, albeit always as outsiders with a broad base of understandings, and so had seven different team members each attend a different group meeting at different times and make observation notes (deliberately with no initial guidelines about what to observe or note). These disparate notes were then analysed for themes. This was done as a group exercise, allowing for some training element as well as a rich exchange of ideas. The preliminary analysis was examined by two team members specifically designated to this project, and an extensive list of themes emerged. This was subsequently used in other group observations in an attempt to understand a broader experience of self-help groups than would have been apparent with only one or two of these initial observations. It might have been even more interesting to have all seven attend the same group at the same time and examine their notes, but this was not possible without significantly changing the composition and, presumably, the process of the group.

Experience suggests the following as a guiding principle: for any researcher we now aim for active involvement in no more than two different research projects. At times, for resource reasons, DART members have had to straddle three or even four projects which is too stressful and dissipates responsibility. It seems harder for those researchers with qualitative leanings to straddle many projects, particularly where there is less distance between the researcher and the researched – a situation which occasionally encourages researcher identification with respondents. This is a problem known in experimental psychology as 'handling your own rat' (a phrase credited to Grice in Frost and Stablein, 1992).

Likewise, the most complex projects that we run, where more than three staff are involved, take a significant additional effort to coordinate and manage than those where the core group is small. There are obvious issues of efficiency but there are also issues of clarity. Some of our most difficult projects and times have been when there are so many different participants with so many ideas that we struggle to find an appropriate pathway; in this environment it is costly to meander too far.

Delegation through a team is both facilitated and difficult! A team culture allows for multiskilling and mutual support but it can make for some difficulties in designating responsibility and, at times, status. In an hierarchical environment such as the health field flat management structures are often not respected. The tensions of teams in this environment surfaces to pose problems. Where the context expects (and sometimes demands) hierarchal organization, teams can be threatened.

Team recruitment

We recruit in many ways: by direct public advertising followed by an extensive selection process; by directly approaching people we know of; people approaching us (sometimes these are applicants for positions we advertise or successful scholarship applicants); or through personnel on collaborative projects. About half of the current staff have been recruited from advertisements. While the resources and effort required to select and subsequently orient staff is considerable, my experience suggests that it often worth it, for example, early this year we advertised three positions: a research assistant, a senior research assistant and a research fellow to take up a PhD scholarship that we had created. We had a total of 93 (55 + 25 + approximately 13) applicants, respectively. For each position we had to write a job description, advertise, create a selection panel, determine selection criteria, read, shortlist, check, interview and re-interview.

There are few undergraduate course components with alcohol and drug content and so few come with a background in the area. We try to encourage them to bring what knowledge they do have and apply it to this area, not to think that there is an esoteric and different body of knowledge that would supplant all that has been acquired.

Gender is always a consideration in appointments to our positions. With ten women and eight men, this team seems well balanced.

Structures to support the research team

Both formal and informal structures have evolved over the past 5 years. These provide the basic communication opportunities, training vehicles and avenues for the generation of new ideas. Our times together are generally positive and enjoyable. The contributions of the various members of staff have been significant in enhancing a supportive, friendly, challenging and active culture.

The formal structures include various project teams and supervision arrangements are not always well implemented. Although new staff and higher degree students have formal arrangements, much eventually depends on the individual researchers seeking out supervision and being active in using the group opportunities. Many of our projects have advisory groups and some involve collaborator meetings.

In addition to these project-specific structures DART operates a series of other meetings, including a weekly journal club, fortnightly seminars and monthly full unit meetings. Generally, all members and students contribute to these meetings and outside speakers are invited in from time to time.

Some 4 years ago we initiated a university-wide interest group (modelled on my own experience of such a group at Colombia University) in this field. The Drug Research and Education Group of the university meets monthly and provides an interdepartmental forum for research and other presentations and an invitation to participants to proceed to a shared meal afterwards. While attendance at each meeting is usually only about 10 or 12, it is a valuable opportunity to meet with colleagues in other disciplines and departments and has connected us with geographers, forensic botanists, criminologists, educators, people from women's studies and pharmacology. About once a year we manage to have an international guest as a part of this programme. It runs on no fees and no funds and is supported by the DART group.

Social and emotional dimensions

Team implies both formal and informal relationships. Both are present and one helps to support the other. Not all DART members are friends; in fact, some might actually dislike one another but retain respect, and while some DART members have formed strong social and personal friendships, others maintain boundaries between their personal and work worlds.

Teams allow a structure for shared management of some of the social and emotional issues that arise in our research. Team members demonstrate enormous mutual care and concern, from personal to research roles, for example support during crises in people's lives; the recognition of the imperatives involved for those of us who live in relationships involving dependents; through to the development of a policy on debriefing through paired linking following field research and interviews which, when appropriately implemented, can significantly reduce stress. It is rare that one team member stands alone, the group being sufficiently large and diverse for a range of alliances to form which cannot always be predicted by former debates.

It is interesting to see that even those in a strong medical research institute, engaging often in laboratory-based research, have a truly human dimension, although in that world it is often not acknowledged (Charlesworth *et al.*, 1989).

Two elements which might seem trivial but which help to cement DART are shared humour and books and a trade in gossip, usually about people and events outside the team, since there seem to be few secrets within!

Teams revealed: the puzzle of an authorship struggle

Although we have a policy that all of those team members who have actively contributed to any project will be listed on publications, and that the originator of the project or idea for a paper should ordinarily be the one to write the first draft of any paper and thus retain first authorship, it is possible for the originator to relinquish this right and allow another member to be first author. This does not avoid all authorship tensions and disputes.

Paradoxically, I have found that the only real disputes have involved my having to lay claim to being included as an author on a specific publication. I do not claim authorship rights on all papers emanating from projects where I am the chief investigator. As someone who has publicly deplored the assumptive worlds where the head automatically claims not only authorship, but first authorship rights whether or not they have been active writers, this was one of my most perplexing experiences. This occurred in a project where the original idea for the research had been mine; I had written the original proposal on my own, I had recruited first one researcher and later a second, and supervised the project for 3 years, spending half a day a week in discussion with the research assistant and a collaborator. I had led the field work and data collection in one of three sites, running groups, consultations and interviewing key players; arranged and supervised a group of students involved in observational work in a range of agencies and led the 1-day session to analyse the results of this effort; written up details for presentations on the project; negotiated access; read and commented in detail on a first draft of the final report, including rewriting some sections and, to my surprise, found that my name was not on the front cover of the penultimate draft of the final report. This was a most painful issue to confront and was not merely a mistake.

The discussion that ensued ultimately involved consultation with the university solicitor and the accumulation of others' experience in such cases. We maintained this at a level of respectful dialogue, but the tension was extreme. My initial request for third-author status was perceived by senior colleagues to be pathetic, yet that was my expectation. I was urged to take action. We managed to resolve this ourselves and now, some 3 years later, are again cooperative collaborators on an extension of that original project.

This clash of beliefs taught us all that justice in research practices can never be taken for granted. The effort involved in resolving this dispute was enormous. A clue to the puzzle might be that this project was an early one for me and one which was midway when I changed from my earlier work place to my current one, with the researchers geographically remaining in the former.

DIFFERENT RESEARCH TRADITIONS AND PARADIGMS

Given the current era and the strength of the debate in the academic world about research paradigms, with a jostling for place in the hierarchy of legitimate knowledge, it is perhaps not surprising that the dominant discourse in DART arises in epistemology and methodology. What is distinctive is that it is occurring within a conservative medical faculty, where the dominance of positivist science remains largely unquestioned.

The medical environment

One of the texts that speaks readily to DART members but would, I believe, be a mystery or regarded with disdain by our departmental colleagues is Guba's (1990) edited book *The Paradigm Dialogue*. We spend less time debating fundamental theoretical issues with our medical departmental colleagues than among our own team, which is disappointing. The reasons for this might be found in the management structure of the department, which encourages the relative autonomy of units, and to some extent in the culture that dominates, a culture which is largely pragmatic rather than a theoretically orientated one.

It is also likely that the arrogance of positivist science remains, for example, on presenting a research proposal to senior colleagues which involved an intense exploratory phase of a study of self-help groups, the response from one was: 'This isn't research because you don't have any hypotheses'.

Sometimes colleagues from other units seek out DART members for assistance in trying to think of ways of answering difficult questions or, more specifically, for advice on qualitative methods. Although maintaining a collaborative and supportive culture, at times we are reluctant to give such quick advice since there is often an assumption that anyone can do qualitative work. As one colleague suggested: 'It's just a matter of doing a focus group, asking a few questions and forming a judgement about the answers, isn't it?'

A lack of understanding of complex alternative research designs, methods of data collection and epistemological debates is associated with a lack of respect for alternative approaches to knowledge development. Those reared in a positivist tradition respond with incredulity when I suggest that qualitative work requires as much or more rigour than quantitative work, is more difficult and necessitates greater immersion in one's work than more traditional approaches.

The other reason that DART is sought from time to time is that relatively few of those with medical backgrounds have any specific training in research *per se*. The influx of other disciplines into health research arises, in part, from this significant deficit. The academic environment for medical researchers has traditionally been laboratory based or through clinical specialties. The areas that our relatively young department is involved in are more recent, and as such are still regarded by many as soft, underdeveloped and fringe activities. There is some research insecurity born of this status among medical members of our department; however (or possibly because of this), we find our GP colleagues can question their knowledge base, the assumptions that they have been reared on, and that they are interested in novelty. They thus represent the friendly end of the medical establishment.

Despite the fact that colleagues in other units look upon DART projects as eccentric and sometimes interesting, they have generally been supportive. An example of this stance is tolerance (sometimes pained) of dress codes that differ from their own: they have adapted to men wearing earrings, occasional tattoos, 'peasant clothing' and long hair. It might seem strange to even mention these elements. The 'difference' of DART is something that I am constantly having to negotiate. The messages are sometimes subtle and often DART is viewed with benign curiosity. Occasionally though, there is a hint of the unacceptable. The position of mediator is one which any team manager knows.

Mixed methods and triangulation

Most DART studies use mixed methods. This arises from the composition of the research groups and from the phenomenon we study. While we sometimes envy those with circumscribed projects who do not struggle with triangulation, the task is to find appropriate ways of bringing diverse data together and to create meaning from them.

Complexities of both analysis and interpretation, and difficulties in finding closure, are common. Appropriate budgeting for these endeavours and management of these budgets is difficult. We still struggle to draw appropriate and necessary boundaries where knowledge is uncertain and the subject of study complex and interactive.

Writing complexity

The dialogue concerning how to write about such work continues. Various efforts have included writing some material from one perspective and a commentary from another; the inclusion of vignettes within the text; visual representation of some elements (e.g. including a map of the venue for a techno rave as a part of a study of hallucinogen use); and sometimes agreement to have one or a cluster of authors write a piece from their own perspective. We are still evolving ways of dealing in writing with mixed methods that arise from differing paradigms and diverse epistemological starting points. Merely mixing this stew is not a workable solution!

One perspective can be fascinating and engage attention; others emerge with contradictory views using alternative approaches; and the sheer mass of information is sometimes hard to integrate. This makes the writing up a larger than usual task, involving data selection, acknowledging and using contradictions, making judgements and, while usually grounding these in evidence, occasionally realizing that they include a leap of conceptual faith.

What we have learned from these experiences is that maximizing mixed methodologies is difficult to do well, requires significantly more effort that a single approach to a phenomenon, and wins us few friends in a theoretically and methodologically conservative environment. It is also stimulating, theoretically challenging and often revealing in health research.

MONEY: A DIRTY WORD

Although the academic espouses interest in the story of our research programme, it is the financial story that underpins and directs our work.

When I started in this environment, on a lower salary than the grant provided for, there were sufficient savings after a year of straddling two part-time jobs, to appoint me full time for the remaining 2 years. With help from the original research assistants I was successful in attracting two other grants and so, after 3 years, I had four research assistants working with DART, one of them a PhD student. At this time roles and responsibilities were clear and each member was working on one specific project. It was the interest, enthusiasm and strength of these early research assistants which in part contributed to my commitment to retain them in the alcohol and drug field and to support them in further research and study. Scholarships were highly competitive in this established university and the only alternative source was further research funding.

Maintaining researchers

Always having at least one project funded for more than a year has provided some stability and continuity. The effort involved to plan, develop, write and submit research grants is known to many. We have been fortunate that some have been funded.

We have also experienced crises. Some result from research funding timetables changing, the unpredictable success in grant applications and straightforward failures. This has produced a somewhat chaotic environment from time to time as we undertake small contract research in an effort to cover funding gaps. Forward planning is complex, since predicting the times when stopgaps will be needed, and uncertain processing times for some of the less establishment funding sources, means uncertainty.

Some of these projects might ordinarily be regarded as more trouble than they are worth. One could certainly question the value of a $3,000 contract when management, liaison, negotiation, contract writing, accounting and supervision are included. If these tasks were costed little real money would remain to do the actual research. In academic environments this infrastructure and management resource is not allocated from such budgets but is mostly squeezed from the head of the research team.

Other pragmatic solutions include seconding one of our team to a project in another organization, which involves collaboration. While these linkages are desirable they come at some cost. For example, one research assistant had some split loyalty. Knowing we were keen to have her return to work with us, she quite reasonably looked to us for ongoing support. We remained her 'peers' and the group to whom she turned when problems emerged in the other environment. As in most cases, this collaboration did not include money for us and so restructuring the project to allow for change was impossible. Hours of personal and professional angst later, the project was satisfactorily completed, but only after confrontations, bizarre confidential communications and a realization that we had inappropriately structured this experience.

In another case, where one of the more senior members of DART worked in another unit part-time to cover a lean period, the issues of ambiguous time and commitment made for considerable stress.

This scramble for resources saps energy and contributes to dissipation of effort. Attempts to maintain quality research are sometimes compromised. It is difficult to let promising, interested and loyal staff go, but in more recent times we have turned down many small projects in an effort to bring more focus to our programme. This has meant losing some promising staff where significant training and development had already been invested. There is some solace in providing better-trained researchers for others' projects, but it is hard to lose them.

Over the past 2 years we have had staff who have successfully achieved scholarships or fellowships. These now support four members and we have created a fifth from a grant which was insufficient to provide for a senior salary for 3 years, but which allows the creation of a PhD scholarship.

Supporting researchers

Administrative and secretarial support is as thin in our department as it appears to be elsewhere. We have access to a small, somewhat geographically remote, general pool for this support and this effectively means that we do it ourselves, except for some assistance with accounting. As technological support increases it seems more and more difficult to obtain human support.

All keyboard tasks have been shifted to the research and teaching staff, telephone answering is increasingly managed by message machines, and physical structures that separate different clusters of staff make for alienation and stress. The new technologies of e-mail, the internet and so on add to the tasks of the day and change working hours to a 24-hour clock. Over time we can become as immune to reading e-mail messages as we eventually became to the apparent urgency of faxes.

Research funding anomalies and complexities

The usual policy of funding sources is not to fund the chief investigator. In our environment this means two things: first, all of the projects have to be carried by the person who has some independent funding, and who is not (technically) dependent on the grants themselves. This contributes to overload for many who find themselves heading teams where all are employed on project funding. Secondly, it leaves both projects and personnel constantly vulnerable. The soft money track is difficult even in a time of plenty, with shifting priorities and increasing competition.

The formulae for allocation of additional research infrastructure in Australia means that the research strong who have been successful in attracting grants are given more. The rich get richer and the poor try to become superhuman. While DART receives a very small share in the departmental support allocation (approximately $700 a year to assist DART members to participate in local conferences), this is the first year we have received input from elsewhere in the university and it has come from a quaint source: the University Floral Society has chosen our research team as the recipient of its annual monies for 1994! This group of (mostly) elderly women who meet monthly and are involved in the provision of floral decorations for a variety of university functions, made contact with me after we were apparently suggested as a worthy project. This will provide us with a welcome $2,000 at the end of the year and represent the majority of our discretionary money.

Research funding priorities

Although DART was initiated during a time when alcohol and drugs were a trace flavour of the year (never having a large allocation, but in comparison with previous times a significant increase), we have survived long enough to experience the dwindling of interest or shifting of priorities to apparently more important economic imperatives.

This has been accompanied by a move away from funding for investigator-initiated research to increasing commissioned and contract research.

There are new and different competitors in this territory and it is harder to sustain a consistent research focus. Old assumptions about university-based research persist among funders, for example, when discussing the amount of money we had nominated in a rare attempt to tender for research, we were asked how we came to put in for items such as equipment and administrative support. Further exploration revealed that this was seen as legitimate for a commercial research group, but weren't we from the university?

In this environment retaining network connections and staying close to the shifts in political concern in order to anticipate and, if possible, influence the next flavour of the year can be vital. Even at the micro level this conflict is manifest. Conferences and meetings become network and lobbying opportunities and it is rare for some to find the time to listen to the papers being presented.

Being used or just learning?

There are times when business and research practices join, sometimes reaching their lowest common denominator and at others trading status for other rewards.

On more than one occasion DART has been asked to develop a research proposal for a specific inquiry. These requests often emanate from government (at various levels), and occasionally they are subsequently further developed through ongoing consultation and then funded. We have also had the experience of investing considerable resources in developing a complex and sophisticated evaluation research proposal to examine the effectiveness of correctional-based alcohol and drug treatment services, only to find that we have subsequently been asked to tender for this research and sent our own draft document as the tender brief! Beware the uninitiated!

An even more seductive caller is the World Health Organization. DART was invited to participate in a WHO study which appeared to provide an opportunity for international collaboration and a wider forum for our activity. It was also a project of some intrinsic interest, since it aimed to develop a way of describing patterns of drug use internationally. On discovering that the endeavour was to design a standard instrument for the global population, our concerns about flawed logic having been already expressed, we agreed to pilot the instrument in our city. Because of our considerable concern about appropriateness in diverse cultures, we arranged for a colleague to seek advice from a remote-living Aboriginal group of women. Their feedback led us to recommend that this was an unworkable endeavour, notwithstanding our considerable efforts in randomly selecting some 200 households, distributing and administering the questionnaire; writing a detailed report on the instrument itself; and issues associated with its administration in the city. The project was sensibly ended and so too was our future with the WHO! It cost us considerably more than the approximately $5,000 allocated and we put the extra effort/resources down to experience and learning, which was subsequently used to conduct a survey of women in the general population about their experience of alcohol.

Payment of subjects

We generally wish to pay people who share their time and experience with us. Sometimes we can and sometimes we cannot. Our experience suggests that money can make a difference in recruiting subjects for some of our projects. While ethics committees have raised questions about giving money to 'drug addicts', we have been able to persuade them that this is just.

A related matter is paying a subject to recruit other subjects. We have found that this has been one of the most efficient uses of our scarce resources, but we have had to monitor the process carefully and run training sessions with our paid recruiter after checking on his understanding of informed consent. The values and rules of conduct in the drug subculture can be quite different from those of researchers.

ETHICAL ISSUES

All who are engaged in human research today share anecdotes of the substantial hurdle that ethics approval has come to mean. From a base of concern for subjects and researchers, and increasing efforts to screen, monitor and protect the interests of the researched, have sprung tiers of bureaucracy which can be a mere step along the way or, in some cases, the most difficult step in the whole research endeavour. Our experience spans this spectrum.

Some of the issues associated with the research ethics committees we have worked through include composition (with quasi-legal processes and considerations being carried out by those with limited training in either ethics or law) and clarity of purpose, where there sometimes appears to be confusion between consideration of the ethical aspects of the research and the appropriateness of the methodology or research design that is being used. While it can be argued that methodology is the business of ethics, since one should not involve subjects unless the effort is meaningful, appropriate and valid, these aspects of ethics committees are messy.

I should also say that ethics committees can at times be supportive. We have had occasion to seek ethics committee approval for some unusual procedures, e.g. studying an organization and its members which is, by definition and constitution, anonymous and where members are only ever known by first names, the development of a procedure which could allow for the recording of informed consent without knowing or recording the subject's name produced the novel idea that we tape the subject's consent (allowing for some potential linkage of the voice to the individual but without using names).

Ethics or law?

A more problematic issue arose in another exploratory study of hallucinogen use, where, soon after starting observation work and initial interviews, the researcher drew my attention to the possibility of being involved in environments where illegal drugs were being used, and asked about appropriate behaviour should he be included in a police bust or inquiry.

It is tempting to suggest that, had we known then what we know now, I might have suggested we take the risk. Since this would have been irresponsible, we sought advice from a series of people, including a Deputy Commissioner of Police who had been interested and involved in research in our area for some time; a private solicitor who had represented many people in drug-related matters before the courts; a professor of criminal law in our own university; the university solicitors (with regard to both issues of criminal or other liabilities as well as questions of insurance cover for researchers engaged in such work); other researchers in both Australia and overseas; a professor of criminology; a senior lecturer in the law faculty with experience in the ethics of research (in health areas in particular); clinical bodies' ethics committees; and colleagues and friends. Most of these consultations started out as informal but eventually became formal. Letters were sent to the police, the Attorney General's office; peak professional groups in the alcohol and drug area; and the University Ethics Committee.

The story of this conundrum requires its own chapter. It was filled with complexity; differing and contradictory legal and other opinions; extraordinary frustration; some tentative acting out; and a halt to the project. All DART projects where we were inquiring about illegal activity were also halted, as there was a concern that it could be an offence to be in possession of knowledge of criminal activity and not pass this on to the police, something which our research ethics and promise of confidentiality precluded. This included projects where we had incorporated standardized research instruments which had been used elsewhere to determine the degree of dependence on drugs and associated behaviours, e.g. questions about major crime as well as questions about the use of illegal drugs.

Thinking that this was merely a glitch to which we would find a solution within a a week or two, I suggested that the researchers involved prepare a background paper on the issue, canvass others' opinions and experience, and we would work it out.

It is sufficient to say that this research was held up, with no data collection allowed for 6 months, but at no time was it apparent that it was going to take this long to resolve. Each week saw a new opinion, a new angle on the interminable debates among amateur and professional lawyers. Efforts to gather support from colleagues elsewhere met with mixed success. Some had enormous sympathy, having contemplated this minefield before but usually deciding to take what seemed like a minimal risk. Others were most concerned that this might become 'public'. We discovered colleagues in many places engaged in collecting information about illegal activity who were worried that if our experience was to be generalized, their project would also be threatened. They wanted to support us but were sometimes explicitly asking us to hush the whole thing up; urging us to sacrifice this one project in order to allow others to proceed unquestioned. Other academic colleagues were outraged and active in seeking opinions from international researchers about these matters.

Strategic considerations were focused on the best way of unblocking the system to allow us to proceed. One of the major tensions was whether to continue to work this issue through the proper channels and/or to seek external publicity to push for decisions and action. This tension was constant both within DART and between DART and other parts of the department and the university. While proceeding predominantly with the formal routes of communication in the university, we agreed to other initiatives.

A decision to allow for a limited and carefully written public statement of our dilemma in a news sheet distributed by the Australian Drug Foundation, led to two regional newspapers giving it some publicity, including an interview with the research assistants involved, with the headline 'Legal fears hold up drug use research' (*Ballarat Courier*, 29.3.94) and an opening sentence reading: 'An academic researcher studying illegal drug use has resumed his research project after a 6 months' disruption while his university sought advice on whether he was risking incriminating himself'. The researcher, when subsequently interviewed by the paper, went on to criticize the ethics procedures of the university, thus requiring more mediation and advocacy from me!

We had formed a view early in this process that the university would need senior legal advice, since our efforts to clarify matters of law suggested a complex and contradictory arena. Legal questions included whether being in possession of information about illegal activity and not passing it on could itself be in breach of the law; the risk of a criminal charge of contempt of court if the researchers refused to supply information to the court if asked; and the issues associated with the employment contract and employee cover for work-related injuries (if it could be found that he was involved in illegal activity at the time of the accident, this was said to be void).

The answers were probably all positive. Eventually the issue was apparently resolved by the university seeking a Queen's Counsel opinion and, although we have not been given a copy of the written opinion, we were granted approval to proceed. By this time, very little of the original budget remained and we had only a small handful of interviews. It is a credit to the enthusiasm of the researcher involved that the study was completed, with fewer subjects than originally planned for but still a substantial report written. The personal and professional costs of the exercise were, however, considerable. There would not have been a week where this problem did not have some active manifestation, whether it be a new legal opinion or differing interpretations of responsibility between the research team and other parts of our department, or merely the effort required to sustain a group of researchers who were eager to get out and get the data but prevented from doing so by the conundrum.

The option of terminating the researcher's employment was not seriously entertained. There was a constant sense that this was something which would soon be sorted out (and since there were many equivalent projects being conducted in our own state, elsewhere in Australia and overseas, it seemed silly to think that we would not proceed). The researchers involved were keen, and had either come with a rich background in this research or had been trained in the team to do these research projects, so there was already considerable investment in them. They busied themselves with additional literature work, setting up supportive structures within DART, meeting with colleagues about these issues and thus shifting their focus from researching a drug-using phenomenon to one involving researching the ethics and legalities of research in this area. Human consideration made it difficult to suggest laying off staff, and each hurdle that appeared eventually strengthened our resolve to persevere.

In an attempt to utilize this experience for future researchers, we are currently writing it up for a range of audiences and have plans for a university forum on the topic. As we approach this, support is emerging from others who are starting to confront some of the same issues. It does not feel quite as lonely now as it did a year ago.

The irony was that for one of these halted projects we had consulted with a professional ethicist prior to writing the ethics proposal. This was a complex project, involving as it did the study of an organization where membership was 'anonymous'. We had been asked to rewrite it, being told that we had included too much detail and it was too academic! On doing so, it, like the other projects involved, had been approved some months earlier.

Elusive substances

In another study a somewhat different legal issue arose. Involved in a descriptive study of khat, a drug new to Australia, the research team had included in the original proposal the possibility of tracking and studying the distribution, use and usual practices of a group of users of the drug following importation. One of the reasons the Commonwealth Department had commissioned this research was to investigate both its appropriate legal status and the usual practices associated with its use. It soon became apparent that the group who used this drug were predominantly east African immigrants and refugees, and that due to the short half-life of the active constituents after harvesting, it was imported by air from time to time and used in a fairly confined group.

The research group had developed access and agreement from such a group to observe the use of the drug and had anticipated this in the original proposal which had been funded. The Commonwealth Government was responsible for issuing licences for transportation, but when it came to the concrete request the drug's uncertain legal status in our state prevented this. Thus, the study had to be done with no access to the drug itself and no direct observation of its use. The team was told that there was a khat plant in the local botanical gardens, but that all of its leaves had been stripped. A midnight raid was never executed!

Ethics of funding

It is difficult to indicate the extent of conflict involved in seeing a research team eke out an existence in an environment where there are bodies eager to support us with money which we have decided we cannot ethically accept. Perhaps naive, but at least still honest, we see others accepting that which we have shunned and go on to much more supported research environments with substantial outputs.

In this area, tobacco and alcohol money is potentially plentiful. This has led to considerable angst within my own academic environment, where colleagues have been known to flirt with these sources. My only compromise has been to participate in forums where research priorities and issues have been discussed and where the delegates have been supported using alcohol money. I have never knowingly accepted tobacco-linked money as a researcher, although I grew up on a tobacco farm and it was this that predominantly supported my family and hence my education.

Multiple roles and the politics of research

Maintaining a research team requires multiple roles. I have already implicitly covered many: mediator, negotiator, advocate, counsellor, teacher, supervisor, mentor, interpreter, colleague, friend and critic. Both internal and outside roles are necessary to sustain research and they often compete for attention.

Outside roles become essential for survival as credibility relies on being known and available. A few may achieve this through their publication record, but the health field has at Last two important audiences: a community of researchers and a world of practice and service delivery or policy development. To this might be added clients and patients, funders and the general community.

This role includes significant meetings, negotiations, liaison, community effort in worlds that span researchers (sitting on research advisory panels, acting as reviewer and referee, thesis examiner and occasional adjudicator in research-based disputes), community service delivery advisory panels, government policy and programme planning groups, peak bodies in the field at both state and national level. I also work on writing grant proposals together with the research team. These activities take time, but it is only those who have secure positions who can afford to ignore these roles.

Sustaining enthusiasm and finding solutions to theoretical as well as practical problems makes for little or no routine in a day. Arriving at work to find that almost all of our computers have been stolen (and subsequently taking 8 weeks to replace them); receiving a phone request for information for a ministerial briefing; seeing a deadline date looming; talking to a student who is ill or struggling; reading and joining the weekly staff seminar; dealing with a persistent journalist eager to have a drug story or trying to interest another one in issues about women and drugs; reading for the next meeting and staying sane: all take tenacity, good health and personal and professional support.

Access

The main reason for sustaining these roles is that they are intrinsically linked to issues of access in our research. Access is never a given and is not constant: continual negotiation is necessary, even after early agreement has been reached. In our environment, much of what we study is either often deliberately hidden or covert and/or the subjects are at best suspicious or resistant: for example, following up drug users; evaluating programmes where staff are usually resistant to having their own practices or programmes examined, even when they are keen to have an evaluation product; seeking to explore and describe the way in which welfare agency clients might be experiencing early alcohol career difficulties; and where there is a strategy to introduce the welfare sector to possible earlier interventions when all they want is for someone to take away all of their late-stage dependent and problematic drinkers to a specialist facility and thus rid them of this group. As others have written, gaining access is a complex business (Burgess, 1991), so different from where you go into a situation because they really want you there, finding out about things that they are interested in.

FROM RESEARCHER TO MANAGER

I cringe as I write the word 'manager', surrounded as I am by undermanaged projects. Over the past 5 years my own task has increasingly become one of research facilitator and manager.

Delegation is usually suggested as the solution to overload. This is difficult in an environment where every staff member is on a very limited tenure. The longest commitment in the team is my own, having taken up a 5-year contract almost 3 years ago when I resigned from my previous tenured position in order to continue in drug and alcohol research, at a time when DART was midway through two projects. The next most senior member of DART has been maintained on contracts varying between 1 and 9 months for almost 5 years, and the majority of the other members have contracts which last for less than 6 months. This has been the situation since we began. In this state it is difficult to ask others to take on commitments that require follow-through, community roles where continuity is often critical, and where even the understanding necessary is limited.

Annual requests for extra training in management and administration have produced no training: there appears to be little acknowledgment that middle managers might benefit from it. Heads of departments get some; administrative line staff get some; but those of us who are notionally in academic positions do not (at present, anyway). In the light of the prominence of money matters in my world, requests to have some input on budgeting and accounting are particularly poignant.

At the end of the day

Like others, I have discovered the loneliness of heading a research team. The decisions that have to be made and the times late at night in the empty office are sometimes gladly interrupted by the arrival of a DART member dropping back into work.

At the end of the day, I am the one that has to pick up on unfinished business. In an environment where research assistants are on relatively low pay and their future uncertain, they sometimes manage to retain some integrity which I want to support. This usually means that if there is a 'dirty job' to be done I have to do it, for example, a project involving the evaluation of a health promotion activity included conducting a series of focus groups. These were planned and conducted by me with another research assistant. The funding for this project was limited and the assistant involved moved to another project immediately after the interviews were done. On talking with a research student about his interest in assisting with the analysis of these, he indicated that since I had only 5 days' funding available to pay for this, he did not want to do it as it would not allow enough time to do it 'properly', i.e. maximizing all data, adapting and developing an appropriate analytic framework and tools, and writing this up. He was right; 5 days would not allow that. In the end the original research assistant and I had to do it in two long nights!

Success?

In this environment it is difficult to know what constitutes success. In the research domain, the formal criteria that are used which appear to become increasingly mechanistic include activity indicators such as research out-puts (publications, presentation to conferences, citations); successful grants (with different values depending on source as well as total amounts); the qualifications of staff; the number and nature of higher degree students (especially PhD candidates) and the like. In teaching we are the subject of increasing student evaluations using fixed global ques-tions. Community services activity is regarded ambiguously. It is likely that it is seen mainly as an adjunct to the other activities; necessary to maintain resources and credibility; helpful in keeping the university rele-vant; and providing some input to policy and programme debates, but certainly difficult to assess.

On all of these criteria DART has done well. We have been successful in attracting significant research grants; we now have a number of higher degree student scholarships; we have a reasonable publication record; we are represented on a number of the major research advisory groups in the country. We do not have strong international links but these are develop-ing. Our teaching is well regarded.

Notwithstanding the importance of these indicators, perhaps the strongest achievement has been in creating an intense, stimulating envi-ronment for new researchers, where talk of ideas and challenge is impor-tant. Mentorship appears to be thin in universities today: it goes at the expense of more money-driven activity. I may be heading for extinction in this environment, where the strongest rewards are in the feedback from fellow team members and there is always the danger that it distracts energy from the dominant imperative – reinforced more each year – to constantly win funds.

Frost and Stabelein (1992), in reviewing various exemplary research projects and commentaries on these, conclude: 'At the end of the day per-haps the most useful thing researchers can do is to take their eyes off the intended positive impact of their work, at least initially, and do work because it is intrinsically interesting and important to themselves and their vision of the field.' We try.

I ponder what the natural lifecycle is for a team such as this. I recognize that we have pursued a mission of knowledge building and mentorship when we have only been funded to do specific research projects. At times I wonder if a private setting where entrepreneurial, individualistic research is expected would really be different. I have concerns that the drive to find funding can distort methodology and research findings. DART has done a number of things that we are not clearly paid to do: we talk; we reflect. We know that doing research is not a linear process. It is a messy business, involving contradictions and requiring persistence, and it is demanding. It is also stimulating and rewarding and can help to make sense of the complexities of health and the human condition.

POSTSCRIPT

This has been the hardest piece I have ever written. To write about the pleasure and the pain of running a research team has been most poignant during a month when it has been necessary to give two excellent research assistants a month's notice owing to a shortfall in funds, related to the halt in data collection earlier in the year and when they are only halfway through the project.

We are now halfway through my 5-year contract. One of the ironies of writing this chapter is that by the time it is published DART may no longer exist. For the past year I have been required to work as acting director of Turning Point, a newly established alcohol and drug centre, as the government-funded part of my salary. This necessary involvement with these developments, the devolution of government services to the private and non-government sector, and a decreasing political interest in the drug and alcohol sector within a context of already shrinking resources for research, has meant personal and professional demands which are proving to be counterproductive to my availability to lead DART properly. Perhaps a new DART will develop in this new context which will provide the stability and critical mass that we have lacked.

REFERENCES

Burgess, R.G. (1991) Sponsors, gatekeepers, members, and friends, in *Experiencing Fieldwork. An Insider View of Qualitative Research*, (eds W.B. Shaffir and R.A. Stebbins), Sage Publications, Newbury Park, pp. 43–52.

Charlesworth, M., Farrall, L., Stokes, T. and Turnbull, D. (1989) *Life Among the Scientists*, Oxford University Press, Melbourne.

Frost, P. and Stabelein, R. (eds) (1992) *Doing Exemplary Research*, Sage Publications, Newbury Park.

Guba, E.G. (ed) (1990) *The Paradigm Dialog*, Sage Publications, Newbury Park.

Jackson, J.K. (1954) The adjustment of the family to the crisis of alcoholism. *Quarterly Journal of Studies on Alcohol* **15**, 562–86.

Orford, J. (1975) Alcoholism and marriage: an argument against specialism. *Journal of Studies on Alcohol* **36**(11), 1557–63.

Whalen, T. (1953) Wives of alcoholics: four types observed in the Family Service Agency. *Quarterly Journal of Studies on Alcohol* **14**, 632–41.

CHAPTER 2

Moving beyond biomedical research in health education

Derek Colquhoun

INTRODUCTION

At a time when academics in universities are being coerced to fall into line with the 'publish or perish' mentality, and when conditions of employment are constantly being eroded at the expense of bureaucratic and administrative exigencies, it is easy to stop persisting with (seemingly) endless cycles of writing grant application after grant application. There are of course many reasons why academics continue to apply for research grants in what are increasingly difficult odds. Quite often the pursuit for knowledge in its own right is marginalized or even forgotten because of the need to be seen to be bringing monies into a school or department, or even simply to maintain conditions of work which have been subjected to the administrative and bureaucratic forces of attrition and domination.

In this chapter I will suggest that the odds are still stacked against the researcher in health education, not just because of the increased competition for funds but also because the competition is dominated by a natural science model of research which serves to marginalize attempts to engender alternative, socially based research programmes. Using a personalized account, I will identify this dominating discourse in health education research – a discourse of biomedicine which is driving the agendas of most research agencies in the health area, and which is frustrating many academics who are disillusioned with positivism and the failure of the natural science model of research to explain and account for many of our health problems and inequalities. After relating some of my experiences with various funding agencies I will outline my own research programme, which I find extremely useful and which is based on what Giroux (1988) calls 'cultural politics'.

BIOMEDICINE AS A DOMINATING DISCOURSE IN HEALTH EDUCATION RESEARCH

In February 1990 the PHRDC (Public Health Research and Development Committee) of the National Health and Medical Research Council funded a weekend workshop for health social scientists, which I attended. The workshop's purpose was to discuss the contributions which health social scientists from a range of disciplines, including anthropology, economics, education, history, political science, sociology and social demography, could make to health research in Australia. There were researchers at the workshop who displayed a vast knowledge of the diversity of health social science research. However, a recurring theme and problem for the group was the agreed dominance of 'a paradigmatic preoccupation with a positivist model of science which is rejected by many social scientists as the sole route to knowledge' (Daly and Willis, 1990). In particular, researchers working on theoretical concerns or adopting qualitative research methods felt they were being marginalized for funding, or at the very best having to work in a hostile and unsympathetic research environment. Put simply (and crudely), biomedical researchers (those with a medical background who adopt quantitative research methods) in areas including clinical medicine and science, biostatistics, epidemiology and preventive medicine, were attracting the most money and health social scientists were having to engage in reduced or unfunded research. It appeared to these researchers that studies which included observation, prediction, objectivity, intervention, manipulation and generalizability were getting preference in the funding stakes. This concern has been echoed recently by Hall (1994), who suggests that the 'gold standard' of research in the public health area is the randomized controlled trial. However, Hall identifies the problems of the randomized controlled trial, where:

> ...the study group selected for inclusion is carefully proscribed to maximize the ability of the trial to show treatment effects...patients with co-morbidities or those who are unlikely to comply with the treatment are regularly excluded, as are the elderly, those who have poor understanding of English, are frequently women...researchers select 'black and white' cases, although real patients come in varying shades...the patients who turn up are frequently sick with other conditions, old, frail, and female! Trial patients are rarely typical, and consequently trial results are not generalizable to clinical practice.

She continues to suggest that 'it is commonly reported among public health researchers that non-experimental methods are regarded as 'soft' while qualitative methods are regarded as decidedly squishy' (p. 1).

MY OWN EXPERIENCE

I arrived at Deakin University, Geelong, Australia, as a neophyte researcher in health education. I had always enjoyed research and found the work for my PhD particularly stimulating.* In the 5 years that I have been at Deakin I must have applied for at least 20–30 grants, ranging from ARC (Australian Research Council), PHRDC, university and faculty internal grants, Diabetes Foundation of Australia, Victorian Health Promotion Foundation and so on. I have been particularly persistent in applying to the National Heart Foundation of Australia (NHFA) for research support, especially since the NHFA has a strong presence in schools through professional development services to teachers and the production of curriculum packages such as *The Heart Health Manual*.

Each year I have diligently applied to the NHFA for what they call 'grants-in-aid-education', the funding for which comes largely from the skipping programme 'Jump Rope for Heart' (JRFH), in which many children, particularly in primary schools, participate. Some of my early research as a postgraduate student involved examining the physiological benefits of children participating in JRFH programmes in school, and so I felt I had some sort of affinity with the NHFA. As I was to discover, this was misguided! After 3 years of unsuccessful applications I decided I needed a different approach. I called them and asked for a complete list of all the grants awarded for 1993. Table 2.1 summarizes the distribution of those grants to education and non-education areas (as defined by the National Heart Foundation of Australia), and is a graphic illustration of how biomedical research dominates the funding in the health area.

Table 2.1 Distribution of research grants-in-aid-education in 1993 by the National Heart Foundation of Australia

	Number of grants in 1993	Total amount awarded ($)	Average grant ($)
Education project grants	2	65 178	32 589
Non-education project grants	37	2 317 540	62 636

I accept that the NHFA is just one example of how research funds are distributed, but I am sure the pattern is similar across the granting agencies. Several issues are raised here. First, the striking difference in the number of grants awarded. Biomedical research has over 18 times more grants awarded than education research. Second, the total amount of money awarded to biomedical research is more than 35 times more than the amount of money awarded to education grants. Third, the researchers who were awarded education grants are actually academics in the community medicine area and not in education. Further investigation of the structure of the research committees within the NHFA indicates that there are no education academics on any of the committees. Fourth, the projects which were funded in education are not education grants at all: it takes a vivid imagination to recognize a text (media) analysis of the reporting of cholesterol and the dissemination of risk reduction programmes for cardiovascular health to general practitioners, as education grants. Fifth, and most galling of all these issues, is that the grants are actually advertised as 'grants-in-aid-education'. Much of the research money available to the NHFA comes from the skipping programme JRFH, which is school based. In effect, the NHFA is taking money from children, their parents and school communities, yet the amount of money channelled back into education is negligible. Yes, the NHFA does produce teacher proof packages and run professional development services, but this does not constitute research into areas of policy, curriculum, school organization, teacher implementation of the packages, children's healthy behaviour and so on. An explanation for the large (and almost obscene when viewed in relation to the lack of awards to education) amount of money awarded to biomedical research is that the number and quality of applications from educators is less than those from biomedics. However, I am actually a research reviewer for the NHFA and I know that this is not the case. Is it worth my while to approve applications for funding when I know that they are unlikely to be successful? Time will tell. (At the time of writing I still had an application pending with the NHFA for a project to begin in 1994. I was not successful.)

My attempts to move beyond biomedical research have been frustrated on many occasions. This frustration is heightened when I examine assessors' comments of my own research proposals. Let me share some of their comments with you. In doing this I am aware of how some researchers view 'the secret garden' of research applications and see the whole process of applying for research grants as a singularly secret, almost covert, activity, the conventional wisdom of which is only available to experienced and senior researchers. I am reminded here of Beyer's (1992) insider–outsider account of life as an academic. My point is that by revealing the 'insider' story of the research application process I may be viewed by some as an 'outsider' for betraying the unwritten code and addressing our research failures. During my time at Deakin University I have endeavoured to pursue case study research working with schools. However, research assessors in the health education area do not like case study research:

Assessor 1: The focus upon two schools is workable but it will limit the generalizability of the data.

Assessor 2:   What will be the characteristics of the case study schools? A number of variables were mentioned...but no details given of the actual case study schools and their characteristics.

Assessor 3:   How were these schools selected? How representative are they of Australian, indeed, Victorian schools? There is an absence of detail, of sample representativeness of the chosen case studies from the proposal. Sample representativeness is crucial if meaningful extrapolation from the data is to influence future practice and policy. In summary, this proposal is worthy of consideration for funding if the proposal is reconsidered to include a combination of qualitative and quantitative measures and sample representativeness is observed.

Assessor 4:   How will changes in policy, curriculum or school community linkages be measured over time? Some of these issues and problems may lend themselves more to quantitative methods.

Obviously I accept that there may have been problems with the applications – no research application can be considered perfect. They are merely snapshots of life, and like all snapshots soon lose their relevance and applicability. Nevertheless, my criticism of the assessors is that they have a preoccupation with measurement, generalizability, variables, quantitative methods and sample representativeness (whatever this is: is there such a thing as a representative Australian school?).

It would be easy to accept this position and continue with unfunded research and acquiesce into teaching and the ever-increasing administrative trivia that exists in universities. I am convinced that it is an exciting time for researchers in the health education area and there are many instances of advances in a variety of substantive and methodological issues. Within a framework of large-scale sociopolitical changes, the health area, whether it be health education, primary health care, health promotion or public health, has undergone significant and radical change (Baric, 1990). Baum (1992) has characterized these changes as shifts from a medical to a socioenvironmental perspective. Simply, the emphasis at the turn of the century was on 'problems', then shifted to 'people' (groups of people, e.g. the elderly, adolescents, women, were 'targeted' for interventions), and finally the recognition of 'settings' or 'places' (hence the term 'the three p's') where health is recognized as intrinsic to the areas of everyday life where we live, work, learn and play.

This emergence of the settings approach has many significant implications for the conduct of research in the health area. For instance, there are many new questions which need to be answered in light of the need for an eclectic approach to theoretical insights which need to be brought to bear on the area. We need to recognize the importance of schools as institutions, for example, with their hierarchical systems of administration, power and influence. Researchers need to broaden their perspectives of health – no longer will we be able to accept purely physical definitions of health: sociopolitical–environmental concerns need to be addressed. New alliances between school subjects are being developed and old relationships are currently being examined and criticized (Colquhoun, 1992). Researchers are currently experiencing a 'dizzying and exciting time' (Lather, 1992) owing to their attempt to grapple with theoretical, epistemological and methodological developments in, for example, areas of feminist and qualitative research, software analysis tools, postmodern/poststructural inquiry and critiques of positivism. Within this context Lather (1992) contends that we are displacing the dominant discourse of positivism with postpositivist paradigms of research which recognize different approaches to generating and legitimizing knowledge. Using Habermas's (1971) thesis as a base, in that there are three categories of human interest: prediction, understanding and emancipation, she suggests a fourth area, deconstruction, which she suggests is the foundation for much of her own research and teaching. Of course there are overlapping interests between these areas; feminist research, for example, could fall into several of the areas, particularly understanding, emancipation and deconstruction.

If we accept, then, that we are moving towards a postpositivist era of research in health education and the potential for research in health education is exciting, then, borrowing heavily from McLeroy and Tones (1991), I would like first to suggest several implications for health education research. Some of these suggestions fall neatly into postpositivist frames of research (understanding, emancipation and deconstruction) while others are a little 'messy' but nonetheless still valuable. Second, after this I will outline my own research agenda in health education which falls under what Giroux (1988) would call 'cultural politics'.

POSTPOSITIVIST RESEARCH IN HEALTH EDUCATION

The possibilities of research in health education are now apparently endless. If we can approach research in a possibilitarian manner, rather than be constrained by the often perceived shackles of biomedical dominance, then I feel we can achieve a great deal. Below is a list of possible research approaches which could be used by researchers to guide their efforts.‡ This is not an attempt to condone any one particular approach, but is simply an array of approaches which the reader may find useful.

1. Research must recognize that health is a dynamic process which is constantly changing. Often research is reported in a manner which does not take into account the temporal dimension of our lives. The 'health career' is often forgotten in our haste to present and publish our findings.

2. When researching health education we ought to take the broader sociopolitical environment into account. For example, the dominance of individualism in the teaching of health education needs to be located within the cultural (and particularly the medical) trend to individualize, atomize and reduce problems to the individual level.

3. As I mentioned earlier, research in health education needs to draw eclectically on a range of theoretical perspectives, epistemologies and knowledge boundaries. This will be enhanced if we can engage in multidisciplinary research of the sort outlined by Daly (1993), who presented the intricacies and politics of a project involving medical personnel working with social scientists.

4. Policy in health education can also be a focus for research. Such policies, ranging from international (e.g. WHO), national, state, regional and school levels can be a valuable source of research. Policies can be read as texts open to deconstruction and reconstruction. Not only that, but the process of policy formation and history can be criticized as well, as for example the inclusion of 'lay' and 'expert' interpretations of health.

5. Postpositivist researchers who are challenging the supposedly neutral and objectified stance of positivist research need to research their own practice in a more systematic and rigorous manner. This will include examinations of relationships between researcher and researched; reflexive accounts of research; narrative, life history and biographical interpretations of research projects; knowledge production and subjectivity; and so on (see, for example, Woolgar, 1988; Stevens, 1993).

6. Research that is seen to be rigorous and applicable to different audiences must be made public. This can take many forms: professional journals, books, seminars, lectures, workshops etc. All too often there are good examples of research being conducted the results of which cannot be disseminated or utilized in a positive fashion by other researchers in the same and/or other fields.

7. Researchers need to be wary of what I call 'rape and pillage' research. This involves researchers collecting data in the field or in different contexts and then using these data to suit their own ends. Participants (and this is related to 5 above) need to be involved much more in the research process. Rather than being used as a valuable source of data, participants and researchers need to establish the research relationships from the start of the research. Issues including reporting, presentation of accounts, confidentiality etc. all need to be negotiated and the research ought to be considered an educative process for all concerned.

8. Research needs to be presented honestly, 'warts and all' (see the first collection edited by Colquhoun and Kellehear, 1993). All too often, research projects are presented in a valoristic and heroic fashion.

Failure is not tolerated. However, failures are important, as also of course are the negotiated criteria for success and failure. Moreover, I would argue that a crucial step in this is the problematizing of methodology. In this regard, Robottom and Colquhoun (1992) contextualize and problematize the methodological issues they encountered in their research, or what they call (after Gitlin *et al.*, 1989) 'the politics of method', in an action research project in the environmental health area. Implicit in this, of course, is the acceptance that to engage in health education research is to undertake a political act which can have consequences and ramifications in many spheres.

I certainly do not want to enter the qualitative–quantitative 'paradigm war' (Abbott-Chapman, 1993), which seems to be prevalent in both education and public health (and has been since the 1970s, particularly in education). Rather, I agree with Abbott-Chapman, who suggests we need a pragmatic resolution approach, and that:

> ...a wide repertoire of both quantitative and qualitative approaches is required in order to establish reliability, validity and generalizability, and qualitative data must be approached with the same rigour as quantitative data...researchers must not only develop expertise in a wide range of both quantitative **and** qualitative methods and techniques but they must also become much clearer about what they are doing the research **for**, i.e. they must become more knowledgeable about political, social and educational contexts of the research and make explicit their own beliefs and values as well as those which gave rise to the research gaining support. [Original emphasis.]

With this in mind it is important to remember what Carr and Kemmis (1986) have to say about education (and thereby the implications for [health] education research). They suggest that first, education activities are **historically** located. Second, they regard education as a distinct **social** activity not merely concerned with the development of the individual. Third, education is intrinsically a **political** act affecting individuals' life chances and wellbeing. Finally, they regard educational activities as inherently **problematic**.

Taken together, the comments by Abbott-Chapman (1993) and Carr and Kemmis (1986) underscore recent discussions in the theoretical, epistemological and methodological debate currently taking place within health education. The dilemma, according to McLeroy *et al.* (1993) is that there is a proliferation of methods, theories and epistemologies within health education and that there is general disagreement over the use of any one method, technique or theory and its applicability to practice. Table 2.2 gives an indication of the models or discourses on health education often used by researchers and practitioners.

Table 2.2 Discourses of health education (modified from French & Adams, 1986 with permission of *Health Education Journal*)

	Behavioural change	Self-empowerment	Collective action
Aim	Changing people's behaviour	Developing people's ability to understand and control their health status	Changing environmental social and economic factors through community action
Models of health	Biological functioning and role performance	Spiritual, physical, mental, environmental and social harmony	Health is a socially defined concept related to individual and group norms
Model of humanity	Rational decision making	Personal fulfilment	People are social animals and rational problem solvers
Model of society	Positivist, hierarchical and stratified	Society is organic, plant or animal-like	Materialist, conflict between factions and various interests
Model of education	Classical humanist	Progressivist: education is about growth and personal development	Reconstructionist: education is an agent of change
Examples	Propaganda: mass media and mass participation campaigns	Lifeskills training. Value clarification	Advocacy. Knowledge and consciousness raising. Community action, pressure groups

The debate has centred on the health education profession's preference for the behavioural change model and the intervention programmes developed within this discourse. McLeroy *et al.* (1993) suggest that the problem with the intervention programmes which are central to this dominant discourse is that they are:

> ...largely independent of the specific health problem being addressed, they ignore what we know about the social production of disease, they are not connected to the field's collective wisdom about what works, with whom, under what conditions and they may lead to inappropriate interventions for the communities in which they are to be used.

CULTURAL POLITICS AND AN ECOLOGY OF HEALTH EDUCATION: A RESEARCH AGENDA

According to McLeroy *et al.* (1993) an ecological approach to health education recognizes the problematic nature of health behaviour. Also, it recognizes that health problems are socially produced and maintained. In addition, an ecological approach uses several levels of analysis, such as the intrapersonal, interpersonal, organizational, community, cultural and public policy. A strength of an ecological approach to health education research is that it acts to synthesize what we know about health problems across a range of levels and not just at one level, usually the individual behaviour causing the problem. Importantly, an ecological approach recognizes the significance of contexts or the settings within which behaviours occur. In McLeroy *et al.*'s own words (1993; p. 310):

> Health education practice should be based on three essential components: first, a clear understanding of the social factors, at multiple levels of analysis, affecting the nature and distribution of a health problem; second, knowledge of interventions, at multiple levels of analysis, that are successful with varying populations; and third, an indepth understanding of the communities, organizations, neighbourhoods, networks and individuals that are the target and context of health education programs.

My own research agenda has been dominated in recent years by critiques of the dominating biomedical discourse of health, particularly as it is manifest through individualism or healthism (Crawford, 1978) in the school curriculum (see Colquhoun, 1991). Of fundamental use in this quest has been the work of Giroux (1988) and his development of the concept of 'cultural politics'. This refers to discourse analysis in three domains: the discourse of production, the discourse of text analysis, and the discourse of lived cultures. Taken together these forms of analysis are particularly powerful for critically examining health education from a postpositivist perspective.

The discourse of production

For Giroux this involves the ways in which structural forces impinge on the process of schooling. For example, how a dominance of technocratic rationality has affected the production of curriculum materials and packages. School community relationships are central to this analysis, in particular the relationship between school, work, the state, the production of knowledge and various vested interests. The discourse of production includes a sensitivity on behalf of researchers to the sociohistorical context of education and a recognition that the curriculum is a product of historical contestation and tension between sub-groups and vested interests. Abbott-Chapman (1993) reminds us that we are in an instrumentalist era of 'corporatist culture', with an emphasis on technical competence and marketable skills.

Central to this analysis is the identification of vested interest groups in health education in schools. Clearly these interest groups come from many areas, including teacher professional associations, quasi-governmental charitable organizations and agencies such as the NHFA, the Diabetes Association of Australia, the Anti-Cancer Council and so on. Of strategic interest is the relationship between various subject groupings within the health area, including the sexuality, drug, physical education and environmental areas. Another concern of this type of analysis is to recognize trends in schooling and in curriculum development in particular. For example, in health education it is possible to investigate the ways in which our lives are becoming medicalized (Kohler Reissman, 1983) and how medicalization is manifest, transformed and translated into curriculum formation and pedagogy. As I mentioned earlier, the discourse of production is concerned with the analysis of the production of teacher proof curriculum packages, which not only influence the way in which children learn health education issues and concepts but, perhaps more importantly, how teachers are perceived in the process of knowledge production. In this approach teachers are often used as cultural dupes and behaviour change technicians to effectively and efficiently implement the curriculum packages designed by experts in the health area.

One research project which has been influenced by the discourse of production is called 'the sociocultural determinants of curriculum in health education'. This project, which builds on earlier research projects, posits that the form of contemporary curriculum in health education is a product of a tension between three conceptual issues and that health has become a symbolic category of considerable importance, expressing a range of notions relating to wellbeing, consumption and normality. A particular view of health as being concerned with the body (corporeal) and individualistic has become pervasive within the new, contemporary health consciousness. The human body has in the past been the property of the biomedical sciences (since the emergence of anatomy as a discipline) and until recently has been ignored as a focus for serious social and cultural research. Biomedicine and scientific medicine have, in the past, defined the body as a machine which needed regular servicing and maintenance. This has meant that scholarly attention has been diverted away from the body as a sociocultural artefact, with its attendant images of morality, normality and social relations and assumptions.

Within school health education and health promotion in general, this focus on the human body has meant that the form and content of contemporary programmes have tended to be factual, ahistorical and asocial. However, the medical profession has recently come under attack from many quarters, including feminists, the poor and socioeconomically disadvantaged, and from the (largely) neo-Marxist sociology of health care researchers. In addition, the healthist (read individualist) orientation of much of what passes as health education or health promotion has been the target of recent developments around the world in the form of the new public health. What is significant to this study is that school Health Education and health promotion have become two sites, among many, where this discourse of healthism is produced, reproduced and legitimated. The school curriculum and health promotion strategies in the broader sphere, then, have become the focus for the tensions and struggles inherent in the definition and redefinition of health and illness, and the changing perception of the role of biomedicine in particular has meant a reassessment of the sociocultural significance of the human body.

It is now well accepted that the curriculum reflects the changing rhetoric of school subjects, which in turn reflects the social function of schooling and the vested social interests that underpin pedagogy, including the form and content of curriculum. What is clear is that the curriculum is socially constructed by the struggle, debate and contestation of particular groups and/or individuals in society, or what Goodson (1992) calls 'the forces of fixity and persistence'. Following on from this it is possible to believe, for example, that the way in which health is perceived in the broader cultural domain forms the context for the presentation of health in the school curriculum. If we accept that curriculum is intertwined with shifts in social values and reasoning outside the school, then it is necessary to investigate the contemporary image of health in society by viewing it through a particular lens which acknowledges an implicit understanding of the social history of health and its particular constituting discourses.

The study complements existing research within the Faculty of Education, Deakin University, and has arisen as an extension to an internal research programme within the university allocated to the chief investigator. This research programme, which was funded with seeding support and which has been informed by the curriculum reform literature as well as the sociology of school knowledge, has tentatively identified, through an analysis of the politics of health education, three related key sociocultural determinants which constitute the regulative discourse of health education.

The project aimed to investigate three school subjects, including health-based physical education, environmental education and VCE (Victorian Certificate in Education) health education in an attempt to locate and identify the broader regulative discourses prevalent in school health education. For Bernstein (1986), regulative discourse is embedded with instructional discourse and is a precondition for any pedagogical discourse which is created by social relations, order, identity and networks. The three sociocultural determinants which I have identified as constituting the regulative discourse of health education include scientific medicine, rationalizations of the human body and, the new public health. Each of these has, in its own way, contributed to the contemporary form of school health education in Australia and in western countries in general. I accept that there may be other sociocultural determinants or discourses, such as holism, which may be dominant in other areas. However, what is of significance is first, the relationship and tension between these sociocultural determinants; second, how they wax and wane over time as social interests and values also wax and wane; third, how they penetrate the school curriculum and are operationalized/marginalized or used as strategic, justificatory or legitimating rhetoric in struggles over the meaning of school health education; and fourth, how new discourses interact with existing discourses. Without detailing these regulative discourses it is clear, for example, that the new public health, which calls for health to be placed on the political agenda, is in the ascendancy. What is imperative is how this emergence is reflected in the curriculum and which teachers' rationalistic tools will be used and employed as it penetrates the curriculum.

In addition, and because teachers and students constitute part of the culture they live in and represent in their curriculum, it is necessary to investigate how their biographical situation influences the form and content of their curriculum. Is it possible, for example, to examine and incorporate aspects of teachers' and students' biographical details into the curriculum? We need an adequate conception of the triad of culture, biography and curriculum. This, of course, is particularly relevant in the area of health education because health as we all know it is a generative discourse through which we attach many of our personal meanings and expressions.

Work in Australia on this topic is limited. Apart from the work of Kirk and Colquhoun (1989), Colquhoun *et al.* (1990), Colquhoun (1989a,b,c), Colquhoun and Robottom (1990) and O'Keefe (1992) there has been no other research in the area to address the problem, specifically related to school health education.

The study has had two related and overarching aims:

● to apply to health education a theoretical framework which identifies the three sociocultural determinants of curriculum in health education and which conceptualizes school subjects as sites of contestation, struggle and tension;
● in so doing to develop a theoretical framework for health education which encompasses the triad of culture, curriculum and biography.

More specifically, the study adopted the following objectives:

1. to examine the influence of the three dominant sociocultural determinants in the production of curriculum;
2. to illustrate ways in which these sociocultural determinants shape and are shaped by curriculum;
3. to investigate instances of refraction, translocation and modification of these sociocultural determinants of curriculum. For instance, to take

an obvious example, how recent work on the new public health is or is not influencing curriculum development and the subsequent teaching of health education;

4. to demonstrate how these key sociocultural determinants of curriculum are congealed in the biographical experiences of teachers and children;

5. to make recommendations to Ministries of Education and the peak subject associations for health education, such as ACHPER (the Australian Council for Health, Physical Education and Recreation) and AAHSC (the Australian Association for Healthy School Communities), around Australia regarding the development of curricula in school health education and the professional development of teachers.

The study attempted to produce theoretical explanations of curriculum and, in particular, school health education, as well as to inform theoretical developments in health promotion. School health education can realistically be called a 'theoretical desert', void of any true social and cultural explanations of behaviour, and therefore, by implication, of curriculum form and content. So far, typical theoretical advances have been firmly rooted in a sociopsychological framework using the concepts of self-esteem, decision making, self-concept and self-control.

Data collection involved policy analysis, historical curriculum analysis, interviews with teachers, lesson observations, text analysis and deconstruction and critical insight into various theoretical interpretations influencing the development of the recent trends.

Discourse of text analysis

The discourse of text analysis includes the analysis of the social construction of knowledge and how meanings presented in texts are contested and contradicted. It involves an acknowledgement that the reader is an active consumer of the text and not a passive recipient of the meanings in it. The reader actively interprets and reconstitutes the text to suit their sociocultural context. Text analysis can be fruitfully used in several areas, including policy and media analysis (Lupton *et al.*, 1993).

As Kohler Reissman (1983) has pointed out most lucidly, the classic example of the social construction of knowledge in the health area is the medicalization of women's bodies. She suggests that women's bodies come under the medical gaze in four major areas: body size and shape (the beauty industry); premenstrual syndrome; reproductive freedom; and medicalization and psychiatry. Kohler Reissman was particularly concerned with the influences of the medicalization of women's experiences on their health. However, she also highlighted how the human body (women's bodies in this case) could be seen as a text, which can be read for different signals, messages, interpretations and so on.

One project in which I have been involved in uses the idea of body-as-text to examine (deconstruct) the ways in which the human body is presented in children's illustrated story books. The central concept behind the project is that the presentation of the human body reinforces the ways in which children think about their body and hence their health. The project is an offshoot of a larger project investigating the politics and dominant discourses in health education. Much of what is taught as health education is dominated by the discourse of healthism – a belief that individual responsibility for health is the sole avenue for improving and maintaining health. Quite often, then, the way we perceive the human body – as an engine needing regular maintenance and servicing – is a reflection of how we think about health. Clearly, healthist notions of self-control, willpower and self-discipline are reflected in the need to maintain and service our bodies. What this does, according to Crawford (1978), is merely support the 'politics of diversion' where the 'real' causes of ill-health, morbidity and mortality are marginalized or neglected.

One major finding so far from this project, which is still in its infancy, is that in children's story books the body is strongly related to personality types and traits. For instance, fat people are often portrayed as indolent, inattentive, often late for meetings, indulgent and so on. The next stage in the research, as I see it, will be to investigate children's interpretations of these story books to examine their constructions and reconstructions of them, particularly as to how the body is presented. It may be the case, as in other research on feminist issues in story books, that children's deconstructions are in fact completely different from those of the researcher, or the meanings presented by the author of the story.

Discourse of lived cultures

All too often researchers in the health sciences present human experience and behaviour in a sanitized and clinical form, stripped of any real in-depth, rich and contextual information. Human experiences cannot be inferred automatically from structural constraints and conditions. An acknowledgement by researchers of cultural politics accepts the complex nature of social and cultural life and uses the dialectical relationship between the individual and the dominant sociocultural conditions as a focus for research and investigation. As part of this investigation Giroux (1985) suggests that we need to develop a discourse about human experience which does not assume that behaviour stems from structural constraints alone:

...in other words, the complexity of human behaviour cannot be reduced to merely identifying the determinants, whether they be economic modes of production or systems of textual signification, in which such behaviour is shaped and against which it constitutes itself.

This discourse which we need to develop Giroux calls the 'discourse of lived cultures'. Building on what Touraine calls a 'theory of self-production' (Touraine, 1977), Giroux asserts that we need to

...understand how teachers (or any individuals for that matter) give meaning to their lives through the complex historical, cultural and political forms that they both embody and produce. (p. 39)

Indeed:

...the discourse of lived cultures needs to interrogate how people create stories, memories, and narratives that posit a sense of determination and agency...if we treat the histories, experiences, and languages of different cultural groups as particularized forms of production, it becomes less difficult to understand the diverse readings, responses, and behaviours that, let's say, students exhibit to the analysis of a particular classroom context. (p. 39)

Giroux's presentation of cultural politics has been particularly influential in my own thinking about the usefulness of large-scale health education interventions, especially with young people in the school setting. I have been in too many schools where the health education curriculum has had no significance or relevance for the students (or any member of the school community). There appears to be a huge gap in what the health experts say we ought to teach and the day-to-day lived experiences of young people. With this in mind, Ian Robottom and myself conducted an Action Research project with young people living in the Geelong (Victoria) region (see Robottom and Colquhoun, 1993, for a more detailed discussion of the project, which was eventually funded). Needless to say, our own interpretations of the concerns of young people were different from those of the young people themselves. We assumed, it would be fair to say, that we thought we knew what young people would be interested in. It is now 3 years since the project began and only now do I feel we are beginning to understand the complex lives of these young people.

I have argued elsewhere (Colquhoun, 1992) that in order to examine the complex nature of healthy (and unhealthy) behaviour a useful starting point has been the triad of context, meaning and behaviour (Figure 2.1).

The relationship between these three concepts is simple, yet often ignored in our haste to define targets, develop interventions, produce expertly designed packages, seek factors influencing behavioural change,

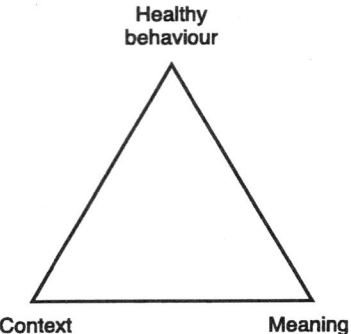

Figure 2.1 The triad of meaning, context and healthy behaviour.

and so on. Clearly, all behaviour occurs within a context and all contexts have meanings associated with them. For example, the behaviour of young people at a party is different from their behaviour at a netball match, or at a shopping centre, or with friends or with family and so on. Studies within a discourse of lived cultures would attempt to investigate what exactly are the contextual issues associated with different behaviours and what are the meanings of the people in the contexts associated with them. Quite simple, yet studies such as these are rare.

Figure 2.2 illustrates how many of the concerns I have raised throughout this chapter have been made operational within a project on 'the health promoting school'. This project, which recognizes the importance of school as a setting for promoting health, is an example of an ecological approach to health education research. First, it accepts the importance of context in determining behaviour. Second, it operates at multiple levels, including the personal, the school, the community and the sociocultural. Third, it examines the trend towards the concept of the health promoting school as a definite social movement with a given sociocultural history within which tensions and contestations are being actively played out. Fourth, it does not take for granted existing (physical) definitions of health and this thing called healthy behaviour. The health promoting school concept encourages a 'holistic' interpretation of health and includes emotional, physical, social and spiritual dimensions. Fifth, the concept of a health promoting school as a setting for improving health is one which can be applied variously to other contexts, for example the health promoting hospital, prison, home, workplace and so on. It is clear that different settings have certain characteristics in common, for example they have boundaries, they often have a hierarchical structure, a defined organizational structure and a range of different social actors within them. Finally, it involves members of communities being actively involved in community health issues, thereby challenging the biomedically reinforced expert model.

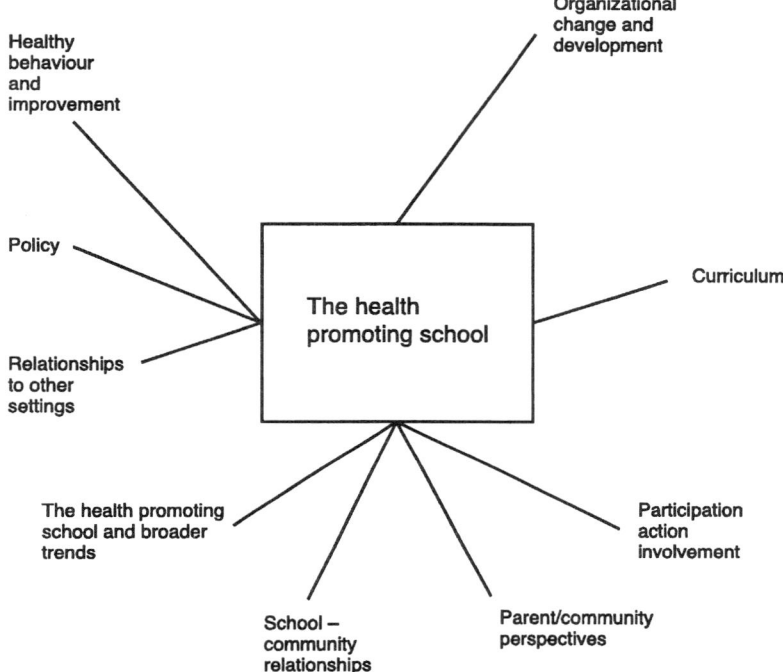

Figure 2.2 Areas of research with the health promoting school concept.

CONCLUSION

In this paper I have attempted to present a personalized account of my own research programme and in particular how it has been influenced by a rejection of a dominating discourse of biomedicine and positivism. I have illustrated my concerns with this discourse by presenting some of my research projects, which I have suggested fall within a cultural politics and ecology of health education. Yes, I have argued, there is life beyond positivist research in health education. However, to fulfil the fruits of that life we need to develop studies which are more creative, responsive and participatory than the studies which tend to dominate our thinking of healthy behaviour and health education. The concept of the health promoting school is one which challenges us to move beyond the traditional biomedical approach to research in health education.

REFERENCES

Abbott-Chapman, J. (1993) Is the debate on quantitative versus qualitative research really necessary? *Australian Educational Researcher* **20**(1), 49–64.
Baric, L. (1990) A new approach to community participation. *Journal of the Institute of Health Education* **28**(2), 41–51.

Baum, F. (1992) Researching public health:behind the qualitative–quantitative methodological debate. Unpublished conference presentation, Methodological Issues in Qualitative Health Research, Deakin University, Geelong.

Bernstein, B. (1986) On pedagogic discourse, in *Handbook of Theory and Research for the Sociology of Education*, ed J. Richardson, Greenwood Press, London, pp. 205–40.

Beyer, L. E. (1992) Transformative tensions: of the inside and the outside. *Journal of Curriculum Theorizing* 10(2), 101–22.

Carr, W. and Kemmis, S. (1986) *Becoming Critical: Knowing Through Action Research*, Deakin University Press, Geelong.

Colquhoun, D. (1989a) Emancipatory health education and environmental education: the new public health. *Australian Journal of Environmental Education*, September (5), 1–8.

Colquhoun, D. (1989b) Health related fitness and individualism, continuing the debate. *British Journal of Physical Education* 20(3), 118–22.

Colquhoun, D. (1989c) Images of healthism in health based physical education, in *Physical Education Curriculum and Culture: Critical Issues in the Contemporary Debate*, eds D. Kirk and R. Tinning, Falmer Press, London, pp. 225–52.

Colquhoun, D. (1991) Health education in Australia. *Annual Review of Health Social Sciences* 1, 7–29.

Colquhoun, D. (1992) Technocratic rationality and the medicalization of physical education. *Physical Education Review* 15(1), 5–12.

Colquhoun, D. and Kellehear, A. (eds) (1993) *Health Research in Practice: Political, Ethical and Methodological Issues*, Chapman and Hall, London.

Colquhoun, D. and Robottom, I. (1990) Health education and environmental education: toward a shared agenda and a shared discourse. *Unicorn* 16(2), 109–18.

Colquhoun, D., Kelly, P. and Stevens, L. (1990) Individualism and school health education: a case study of alcohol education in a Victorian primary school. *ACHPER National Journal* 128, 6–8.

Crawford, R. (1978) You are dangerous to your health: the ideology of victim blaming. *Social Policy*, Jan/Feb, 11–20

Daly, J. (1993) Team research in clinical settings: strategies for the qualitative researcher, in *Health Research in Practice, Political, Ethical and Methological Issues*, eds D. Colquhoun and A. Kellehear, Chapman and Hall, London, pp. 24–36.

Daly, J. and Willis, E. (1990) *The Social Sciences and Health Research*. A report of a workshop on the contribution of the social sciences to health research, PHA, Sydney.

French, J. and Adams, L. (1986) From analysis to synthesis: theories of health education. *Health Education Journal* 45(2), 71–4.

Giroux, H. (1985) Critical pedagogy, cultural politics and the discourse of experience. *Journal of Education* 167(2), 22–41.

Giroux, H. (1988) Critical theory and the politics of culture and voice: rethinking the discourse of educational research, in *Qualitative Research in Education: Focus and Methods*, eds R.R. Sherman and R.B. Webb, Falmer Press, London, pp.190–210.

Gitlin, A., Siegel, M. and Boru, K. (1989) The politics of method: from leftist ethnography to educative research. *Qualitative Studies in Education* 2, 237–53.

Goodson, I. (1992) School subjects: patterns of stability. *Education Research and Perspectives* 19(1), 52–64.

Habermas, J. (1971) *Theory and Practice*, Viking, Boston.

Hall, J. (1994) Health outcomes – implications for research. *Touch, Public Health Association of Australia Newsletter* 11(4), 1–8.

Kirk, D. and Colquhoun, D. (1989) Healthism and physical education. *British Journal of Sociology of Education* 10(4), 417–34.

Kohler Reissman, K. (1983) Women and medicalization: a new perspective. *Social Policy* Summer, 3–18.

Lather, P. (1992) Critical frames in educational research: feminist and post-structural perspectives. *Theory into Practice* **XXXI**(2), 87–99.

Lupton, D., Chapman, S. and Wong, W.L. (1993) Back to complacency: AIDS in the Australian press, March–September 1990. *Health Education Research: Theory and Practice* 8(1), 5–18.

McLeroy, K. and Tones, K. (1991) Editorial. *Health Education Research: Theory and Practice* 7(4), 1–8.

McLeroy, K.R., Steckler, A.B., Simons-Morton, B. *et al.* (1993) Social science theory in health education: time for a new model? *Health Education Research: Theory and Practice* 8(3), 305–12.

O'Keefe, K. (1992) *The History of Health Education in Victoria*. Unpublished Honours Thesis, Deakin University.

Robottom, I. and Colquhoun, D. (1992) Participatory research, environmental health and the politics of method. *Health Education Research: Theory and Practice* 7(4), 457–70.

Stevens, L. (1993) Reflexivity: recognizing subjectivity in research, in *Health Research in Practice: Political, Ethical and Methodological Issues*, eds D. Colquhoun and A. Kellehear, Chapman and Hall, London, pp. 152–70.

Touraine, A. (1977) *The Self Production of Society*, University of Chicago Press, Chicago.

Woolgar, S. (ed) 1988) *Knowledge and Reflexivity: New Frontiers in the Sociology of Knowledge*, Sage, London.

AUTHOR'S NOTES

*My PhD was in primary school health education. It is important to recognize here that I am now writing this chapter after being employed at Deakin University for 4 years, and having been relatively successful (and very persistent with grant applications) in attracting research grants in the public health area.

‡I would not be so arrogant as to suggest that I know all the answers to the problems in health education research. However, I have found these points useful in examining what I consider to be useful research in the area and for focusing on some of the more pertinent issues in my own practice.

CHAPTER 3

Health research and ethnic communities: reflections on practice

Pranee Liamputtong Rice

INTRODUCTION

Most reports about ethnographic field research describe methods and techniques: rarely do they discuss the researcher's social and emotional experiences. Yet in conducting ethnographic field research the social aspect is just as important and is often problematic if not handled properly. Ethnographic field research in the health area is no exception.

This chapter is concerned with the social dimension of ethnographic field research in health. It develops practical suggestions for conducting ethnographic research in some particular Asian and Middle-Eastern communities so as not to jeopardize the researcher's relationship with these communities and hence to allow the research to proceed smoothly. It is based on my personal experience in qualitative health research with several Asian and Middle-Eastern communities in Australia over the last 10 years. It therefore provides a real-world example for those who wish to embark on ethnographic field research in ethnic communities.

The chapter is divided into three stages following the framework used by Shaffir and Stebbins (1991): prior to entering the field; during the fieldwork; and leaving the field and keeping in touch.

STAGE ONE: PRIOR TO ENTERING THE FIELD

How much do we know about the community?

We as researchers need to gain as much knowledge about the community as possible. This knowledge includes, for example, cultural beliefs and practices, values, customs, religion and socially determined behaviours.

The principal view I take is that sensitivity to the culture is good but is not enough by itself. Knowledge of the culture is essential in order to work effectively with members of the community, but this does not mean that we have to come from the same culture and speak the same language. However, if we do it will be invaluable because it will mean that we can understand the issues better and follow them in greater depth. More importantly, we will be able to communicate with the people more effectively. Very often researchers miss a significant amount of subtle detail when they have to work through another person, such as an interpreter. This was my dilemma when I conducted ethnographic studies within communities whose languages I did not speak and where I had to rely on a bicultural worker or an interpreter to obtain information. However, if we are knowledgeable about that community we may be able to pick things up or to follow the issues further, even though we have to work through a third person. Such knowledge can help us a great deal in conducting qualitative health research.

GAINING ACCESS

We need to know how to gain access to the community. The most effective way is to go through the ethnospecific organizations that represent or work for the community. Here we should contact the person who has the highest position in those organizations. Status, authority and respect are important in many Asian countries and these characteristics are still common in the communities now living elsewhere. We need to go to see that person, clarify our intention, bring any paperwork that we have and then ask for help. Usually, if we are clear about what we want to do and ask sincerely for assistance, cooperation can be very good. Once the representative organization accepts us and is prepared to help, it is easy to contact members of the community: they will provide us with names and sometimes even arrange meetings if they have the time and resources.

In the last 2 years I have been doing my field research on childbearing, childrearing and reproductive health in the Hmong community. Prior to entering the community I made several contacts with individual community representatives. With each person I explained about the research project and what benefits I and the community would get from it. I was then able to attend a meeting which was organized on a regular basis for the community members to discuss anything that concerned them. After I had explained my purpose I asked for permission to enter the community and to obtain information from their members. At that time I felt rather anxious. What if they did not grant the permission? What if I were asked to leave the meeting because some of them felt that my presence would have a bad effect on the community? The result was positive, however: I obtained their permission to enter the Hmong community, although there were several conditions attached, the most important of which was the requirement not to cause any harm to the community members. The Hmong have many ceremonies which require certain 'components' that are seen as 'illegal' among Australian people. This might have led to social sanction with the Hmong community. I was asked to promise that when I wrote about the Hmong I must not include any of these aspects in the paper unless they had seen and approved it. Gaining access is, I believe, subject to negotiation between the researcher and the researched. If the community senses any sign of distrust from the researcher, access will be denied.

The best entry is through personal networks, such as contacts with those who have influence in a community, that is, those persons who are well known. In writing about learning to find one's way in conducting an ethnographic research, Fetterman (1991) suggests:

> An introduction by a member is the ethnographer's best ticket into the community. Walking into a community cold can have a chilling effect on the individual ethnographer or in his or her work. An intermediary or go-between can open doors or otherwise be linked to outsiders. The facilitator may be a chief, principal, director, teacher, tramp, or gang members, and should have some credibility with the group – either as a member or as an acknowledged friend or associate. The closer the go-between's ties to the group, the better.

When I was working on a mental health project in a Lao community, I knew a welfare worker who worked for that community. When I asked if he could help me with contacts I received the help I needed. Then when I rang Lao people and explained my research and asked if I could go to see them, before they agreed they normally asked me 'How do you know about me?'. When I explained that I knew them through this mutual acquaintance, they would say 'Ah I see, that is all right. I know that person, he or she has done such and such things for me and my family'. After that, they agreed that I could go to see them at home. So far I have had very few cases where the informants were not at home at the arranged time. Mostly they would be there waiting for me to talk with them.

The right of refusal needs to be addressed here. Although the person was approached through a third party, she would be told about the study and her involvement. She also had the right to refuse to participate in the study at the first point of contact. This process is the same as when we recruit persons from, say, hospitals or other institutions.

What do we know about the people we work with?

When we make contact with respondents we should know their sex, age and their first name. Why is knowing their sex important? I will address this issue in the next section.

Age is important in all Asian countries. The old are respected by the young: this respect appears in the form of how the young address them and a certain behaviour. For example, in Cambodian, Lao and Thai communities when we meet an older person we must pay respect by holding the palms together in front of our chest and lowering our head. Individuals are also addressed differently according to their age. For example, if a Thai lady appears to be older than our mother she must be called 'Pa', but if she is younger than our mother she must be called 'Na'. However, if we cannot guess their age normally we use the word 'Khun', although this word indicates a formal and distant relationship rather than a close one.

If we do not speak the language we should call them by their first name. Most Asian people are not used to being called by a family name and feel more comfortable being called by their first name. We must learn beforehand how to pronounce this because it could cause embarrassment and perhaps sound insulting. Some Vietnamese names are particular cases in point. For example, the name 'Dung' is pronounced as 'Yoong', 'Phuck' as 'Fook', and 'Dy' as 'Dee'. If we address that person as 'Dung', 'Fuc' or 'Die', imagine how embarrassing and insulting that could be!

With my research concerning childbearing, childrearing and reproductive health, part of the project involved Hmong women who had young children. When I contacted a certain woman, I had to ask if she was still breastfeeding her infant because if she was I must enter her house without carrying a bag and not wearing shoes. It is a common belief that strangers who enter the house with a bag and wearing shoes will take the mother's milk away. This is regarded as a serious matter in Hmong culture.

STAGE TWO: DURING THE FIELDWORK (LEARNING THE ROPES)

Look before knocking on the door

Before knocking at the door we must look to see if there is anything attached to it. In the Hmong tradition, for example, a tree branch is hung on the front door to signify the presence of serious illness in the family. In such a situation only the family members are allowed to leave and enter the house: strangers are believed to bring misfortune. Obviously, then, it is important not to enter our Hmong respondent's house if there is a tree branch hung on the front door.

Respect is important

We should be dressed neatly and formally, as this is a way of showing respect. In particular, a female researcher should dress so as not to reveal too much of her body, for example wearing shorts or a miniskirt. Wearing thongs is particularly impolite.

When we enter the house we should take notice of how the person arranges his or her household. For example, taking shoes off before entering the house is very common in southeast Asian communities. One day I went to interview a Vietnamese man at the Housing Commission (Public Housing) flat in Flemington. When he opened the door I noticed a row of shoes placed neatly at the side of the door and he had no shoes on. Consequently, I immediately took my shoes off. Even if the person insists that we can leave them on we should nevertheless take them off, like the owner of the house. This is more respectful.

When we enter the house we should find out if the older family members, such as parents or grandparents, are at home. If they are we should ask to see them and pay respect, or at least greet them. In this way we show that we respect their family.

Very often at the time of interview a husband or the parents of the informant wish to stay in the room. This may present some problems with, say women's health research, particularly, at the point when women are asked about familial relations and women's issues such as menstruation. However, men and older people are highly respected in all Asian and Middle-Eastern societies, and it is not appropriate to suggest that the woman asks them to leave. It would be regarded as improper for the researcher to do so. Whenever this occurred in my fieldwork I would always treat them with utmost respect. They might throw a few answers in for the woman, but I would treat these answers separately in the analysis. I would also ask the woman to confirm the answers. However, very often they did not stay for the whole of the interview: after a few minutes, when their curiosity had been satisfied, they would often leave us alone.

Proper manners

When we are sitting to talk it is considered rude to cross our legs and point the foot towards the person. Looking straight into the eyes is also regarded as impolite: correspondingly she will probably not look at us when talking. This does not mean insincerity or concealment: rather it is more a matter of politeness.

The wellbeing of the informants

One of the ethical considerations in conducting health research is the wellbeing of the informants. One has to be sure not to cause harm to those who agree to participate in the study. However, sometimes the researcher may do the wrong thing out of ignorance. The following is a case in point. In a small-scale society such as the Hmong individuals rely heavily on traditional healers. Some people may become healers by the wish of supernatural beings, as in the case of shamans. However, other healers such as medicine women have to acquire knowledge by learning, and must pay a fee to their teacher. When passing on their healing knowledge, they must also be paid. This payment is to honour the teacher who passes on the knowledge: without it a medicine woman may become seriously ill and perhaps die. This is a serious matter in the Hmong culture.

When I interviewed several traditional healers in my present project I had the privilege to interview two medicine women. Because I had learned what I must do to obtain knowledge from medicine women, I asked them what particular things I should do to prevent ill health befalling them. I was told to perform certain rituals to honour them. On one occasion, the medicine woman asked for $300 as a fee for learning about Hmong medicines. On another occasion I had to prepare a bunch of incense sticks tied with a piece of red cloth, $25 cash and a live chicken. I had to kneel in front of the medicine woman's altar and ask her and her 'teacher' to teach me about Hmong herbal medicines. With this ritual I was then able to acquire the knowledge I wanted. Without the knowledge of what needed to be done before I interviewed the healers, I would have caused ill health or death to some of them. This would have been a disaster for me as a researcher, who had promised not to cause harm to their community, because they still rely on these healers even though they are now in Australia and have more access to western medicines.

Sexual matters

If the project involves discussion about sexual matters we should be cautious. In most Asian cultures sex is regarded as taboo, a formidable matter, not something that should be talked about with other people. However, it is possible to discuss it with a person of the same sex – but with caution. When I worked at a children's hospital a few years ago, I interviewed Cambodian people about their health beliefs and practices. I had to administer the 'Hopkins Symptoms Checklist' (Mollica, 1986). One question in that checklist was about sexual interest or pleasure. I had to say 'Excuse me, I have to ask you the following question in order to complete our questions; please do not feel offended by it or feel that I am impolite'. Then I proceeded and it worked well. This is usually the case as long as we are careful and let the person know that we are aware of and respect their customs.

For the childbearing, childrearing and reproductive health project, I needed to obtain some information related to cultural practices during pregnancy and a period after birth (confinement). One sensitive question is about sexual intercourse during these periods. I again used the apologetic approach before asking the question, and most often the women felt that I understood their cultural norms and values. As a result they were willing to tell me about their practices, often with laughing and giggling.

Here I would like to point out an important issue. Suppose we have to do a project, for example, on AIDS. This requires a person to discuss sexual behaviours and preferences at length. These are extremely sensitive and personal issues since they are tied to social norms, beliefs and values. A sexually active person may be seen as deviant and be frowned upon by community members, particularly the elderly and people of the opposite sex. If we have to interview both men and women, the best way is to have both male and female researchers. In this way neither sex will feel offended by the questions and will feel more comfortable in discussing the issue. Talking about sex with a same-sex person is shameful and embarrassing enough, but it is worse to talk with a person of the opposite sex. The apologetic approach mentioned above still applies even when the researcher is of the same sex.

I also ask for permission from the women even when the topic is not directly related to sexual matters, but anything related to 'women's secrets' such as menstruation and the menopause, since such topics are perceived as taboo. The following is a case in point:

Researcher: I should like to ask you a bit about menstruation, is this okay with you?

Informant: Why do you want to ask?

Researcher: It is related to women's health and having a baby.

Informant: Is it? If we talk about our body having dirty thing, with the Hmong it is the most embarrassing thing to talk about. We do not really wish to talk about it.

Researcher: That is why I ask for your permission before I ask you questions.

Informant: Yes you can ask me, but what do you want to ask?

The above illustrates that when I showed the woman my respect towards her, accompanied by a bit of gentle explanation, she was willing to discuss the issue even though in normal practice it is not usually talked about.

Informed consent

There is an important issue about signing consent forms in some Asian communities. Refugees, for example, have been through many traumatic experiences, one of which was having to sign many papers before they could be settled, particularly if they had already been rejected by other countries. Before we ask them to sign the consent form we should explain clearly that this is something to protect them, not to jeopardize them. Although this is stated in the consent form, and even if it is translated into their language, it is better if we explain it again before we ask them to sign.

However, many Asians and Middle-Easterners are illiterate, even in their own languages, and are not able to read a translated version of the consent anyway. The form should always be read to them by a person who speaks their language, such as an interpreter, or a bicultural worker.

When I and my bicultural researcher were interviewing Hmong women in their homes, I occasionally came across a respondent who felt uncomfortable about signing a consent form. After the bicultural researcher had read out the consent, explained clearly about their participation, and asked for permission to tape record the interview, some of them would indicate that they wished to participate in the study but not to sign the form. Under these circumstances I wrote down on the consent form the respondent's wish and asked the bicultural researcher to witness it.

Another important point is that some women wish to consult their husbands before signing. This was particularly so among Vietnamese and Turkish women, and on some occasions I did not obtain consent because their husbands did not allow the women to participate in the study. However, more often the husbands would be quite happy for the women to have something to contribute to the community, and they even helped their wives to sign the consent form if they were illiterate.

Recording my voice!: no please

In conducting qualitative health research, as with any other qualitative research, it is essential to tape the interview for content analysis. So far I have been able to ask the respondents' permission to do this without much difficulty. Occasionally, though, the respondents might say that they did not like their voice on a tape recorder. However, when I explained to them that it was important to record what they actually said, they consented. Nevertheless, people from some Islamic backgrounds may not wish to have their voice recorded. This was my own experience when I interviewed several Turkish women about childbearing issues early last year (Rice, 1993). A few women, who seemed to be more traditional, did not want me to tape our discussion because it was against Allah's will and therefore sinful. They also said that their husbands would not permit such a thing because a woman's voice should not be heard by strangers. I had to do intensive note taking for the whole 2-hour interview. However, with women who had been in Australia for some time and who spoke English quite well this did not seem to be a problem.

EXTENDING AND RECIPROCATING

During the interview in the informant's home, if we are invited to join the family meal or are offered anything to drink or eat, we should accept. This indicates that we respect their wish. Very often when I went to interview people around mid-morning and finished before lunch time I was asked to stay to lunch with them. It is important not to leave the house as soon as we have finished the interview if we are asked to stay. Indeed, this opportunity is a valid way of observing their way of life, and also offers us a greater chance to obtain further information. Shaffir and Stebbins (1991) argue that the researchers who avoid participating in the informants' activities, when it is possible to do so, and use their participation to make good sense from the research standpoint, lose the opportunity to gain rapport and promote good field relations. The following is also another case in point.

The Hmong grow several herbs in their gardens which play a crucial role in maintaining and restoring health, particularly women's health during childbirth. During the confinement period Hmong women only eat a chicken soup cooked with several kinds of green herbs. These have several functions: restoring the heat lost in childbirth; washing out what may be left in the uterus; stimulating lactation; and restoring strength. Since I was a married woman, many Hmong women gave me the herbs and instructed me how to grow them in my garden in case I needed them in the future. They insisted that I would have to look after my own health by taking the herbs, the same way as all Hmong women do. I do grow the herbs in my garden and have been using a lot in my cooking, even though I am not pregnant.

Many people from countries such as Cambodia, Laos and Vietnam have limited English. Sometimes they will ask us to help in filling in forms, writing a letter to the Social Security Department, 'phoning the school principal about a letter that has come with their children, and so on. Also, children who are in school may ask us to help with an essay or homework. This has very often happened to me when I visit their homes. When I worked as a research assistant at one place I was asked to do these things, but when I raised the issue with the chief investigator I was told not to do it because I was a researcher and not a welfare worker. I strongly disagreed with this view. I believe that if respondents are prepared to give their time to our project and let us learn about their lives, they also deserve a little help from us.

STAGE THREE: LEAVING THE FIELD AND KEEPING IN TOUCH

Charles Gallmeier (1991) writes:

> The process of disengaging from field settings is just as important as the process of gaining entry... Researchers have neglected to include the importance of revisiting the setting and staying in touch with informants after the initial field experience is over.

It is important that we keep our social contacts with the community. By the time we finish our fieldwork, most people in the community will know us. Some of them may even invite us to the family functions such as a wedding, New Year gathering and so on. If we are invited we should go along. This shows them that we are interested in them and their community, not just research or taking things from them.

Even when we are not invited but happen to be in the area we should make an effort to drop in to see them. They normally feel pleased to see us again and this continues our social relationship with them. Sometimes we might bring gifts for them – something from our garden, such as flowers or fruit. Many Asian people grow their own vegetables, herbs and fruit in their home country, and continue to do so if they have a bit of land here in Australia. They really appreciate it if we say that these are from our own garden. We will have lot of things to talk about with them. However, many of them live in flats and have no access to their own fresh foodstuffs. These people will be particularly appreciative of our fresh things.

An important task that keeps many researchers in extended contact with the community they have entered is doing something beneficial for their informants (Stebbins, 1991). There are two examples I am able to provide here. On one important occasion I made several contacts with one of the maternity hospitals in Melbourne and organized for one Hmong woman to re-enter the operating theatre for a soul-calling ceremony, in order to restore her health. She believed that her ill health was due to the departure of her soul during a caesarean operation when she had her last child. After this essential ceremony the woman is now gradually regaining her health (Rice *et al.*, 1994).

When I was editing my book on childbirth and childrearing among Asian mothers (Rice, 1994) I asked one of my informants to be photographed for the cover. In return, the woman and her family received a small sum of money from the publisher (and myself) as well as a copy of the book. Even though the sum was not large it helped the whole family, since they had only recently arrived and relied on social security benefit for survival in Australia. The book would also be a great honour for the family for a long time.

Maines *et al.* (1980) argue that the process of leaving the setting is related to the social relationships and commitments formed during the fieldwork. One may find that one never really leaves the community once strong relationships have been formed: indeed, this has been my experience with the Hmong community.

What is more important about keeping in touch with the field is as Gallmeier (1991) says: 'leaving the setting, revisiting, and staying in touch provide certain methodological advantages... Only by doing so can we make comparisons, improve our techniques, develop better strategies, and learn from our mistakes'. This has been my experience as well. More importantly, I have been able to observe and collect more data when I revisit and stay in touch with the informants. I strongly believe that this should be a mutually beneficial approach for field researchers in health and the people who are generous enough to assist them.

CONCLUSION

This chapter has focused on the social dimension of field health research. I have highlighted the underlying cultural aspects that I, as a social science researcher, experienced while conducting field research, including self-doubt, uncertainty, frustration as well as joy and a sense of achievement. As I have demonstrated, this social dimension is a central feature of the field research process and yet it has received little attention.

> As every researcher knows, there is more to doing research than is dreamt of in philosophies of science, and texts in methodology offer answers to only a fraction of the problems one encounters. The best laid research plans run up against unforeseen contingencies in the collection of data... [However] it is possible, after all, to reflect on one's difficulties and inspirations and see how they could be handled more rationally the next time round. (Becker, 1965)

As Becker has said, our social experiences can be used as lessons for other researchers. My own experiences described here may be used by others who wish to embark on field research in health in communities similar to the ones I describe. Learning about other researchers' experiences and approaches, where very often the formal rules of research have to be 'bent, twisted, or abandoned' in order to meet the demands of the research setting and the personal characteristics of the researcher, is crucial (Shaffir and Stebbins, 1991). It helps to reduce unnecessary errors which may jeopardize the study. If we, as researchers, take these experiences into account we may have some hopeful basis for winning the heart of many Asian and Middle-Eastern communities and maximizing the conditions under which our research will proceed knowledgeably, successfully and sensitively.

REFERENCES

Becker, H.S. (1965) Review of sociologists at work. *American Anthropological Review* 30, 602–3.

Fetterman, D.M. (1991) A walk through the wilderness: learning to find your way, in *Experiencing Fieldwork: An Inside View of Qualitative Research*, eds W. Shaffir and R. Stebbins, Sage Publications, Newbury Park, pp.87–96.

Gallmeier, C.P. (1991) Leaving, revisiting, and staying in touch: neglected issues in field research, in *Experiencing Fieldwork: An Inside View of Qualitative Research*, eds W. Shaffir and R. Stebbins, Sage Publications, Newbury Park, pp. 224–31.

Luangpraseut, K. (1988) Laos culturally speaking. *Journal of Vietnamese Studies* **1**, 11–18.

Maines, D., Shaffir, W. and Turowetz, A. (1980) Leaving the field in ethnographic research: reflections on the entrance–exit hypothesis. *Fieldwork experience: Qualitative Approaches to Social Research*, eds W. Shaffir, R. Stebbins, and A. Turowetz, A., St.Martin's, New York, pp.261–81.

Mollica, R.F. (1986) *Hopkins Symptom Checklist 25: Cambodian Version*. Indochinese Psychiatry Clinic, Massachusetts.

Rice, P.L. (1993) *My forty days: A Cross-Cultural Resource Book for Health Care Professionals in Birthing Services*, Melbourne, Vietnamese Antenatal/Postnatal Support Project.

Rice, P.L. (1994) *Asian Mothers, Australian Birth*, Ausmed Publications, Melbourne.

Rice, P.L., Ly, B. and Lumley, J. (1994) Childbirth and soul loss: the case of a Hmong woman. *Medical Journal of Australia* **160**, 577–8.

Shaffir, W. and Stebbins, R. (1991) *Experiencing Fieldwork: An Inside View of Qualitative Research*, Sage Publications, Newbury Park.

Stebbins, R. (1991) Do we ever leave the field? Notes on secondary fieldwork involvements, in *Experiencing Fieldwork: An Inside View of Qualitative Research*, eds W. Shaffir and R. Stebbins, Sage Publications, Newbury Park, pp.248–55.

AUTHOR'S NOTES

In this chapter the focus of discussion is on Asian and Middle-Eastern communities who are now living in Melbourne, Australia. In particular, those referred to are the Cambodian, Vietnamese, Lao, Hmong, Thai and Turkish people. Lao is taken to mean the Lao ethnics who are the dominant population in Laos. They are referred to as the 'Lowland Lao' or 'Lao Thung' as their habitats usually occupy the low valley in Laos. On the other hand, the Hmong are one group of hill tribes and they are called the 'Highland Lao', and sometimes 'non-Lao'. They live mainly in the mountainous areas. Because both Lao and Hmong come from Laos, very often outsiders refer to them as 'Laotians' (Luangpraseut, 1988). However, the Hmong and Lao are different both socially and culturally. I personally prefer to refer to each group separately.

An early version of this paper was used as a working paper for consumer advocacy for the Health Issue Centre in Melbourne in 1994.

I should like to thank Lyn Watson, who provided useful comments and insight in the preparation of this chapter.

CHAPTER 4

Close to home: qualitative research with people with HIV/AIDS

David Stephens

No one will go far wrong who remains in close touch with and seeks to understand a body of concrete phenomena'. (George Homans, 1970)

There is a particular irony for me in Homan's statement. It is in the certainty that 'no one will go far wrong' – a sentiment that I also felt during my research. This is because I was doing quite a lot of research on a topic on which it would have been difficult for me to get any closer to the phenomenon I was seeking to understand. I refer to some of the issues that I faced in researching a group of which I am a member. My account is a personal one and discusses how my proximity to the questions I analysed affected the research and how the research affected me. Even though I was intimately acquainted with the subject matter the issues raised did not rely solely on this. They are part of broader methodological debates concerning the politics and practice of research. My closeness to the subject simply made this more acute.

I was diagnosed as having HIV in 1987. Between 1991 and 1994 I conducted research on HIV and AIDS, a requirement for the completion of a Master of Health Studies degree at La Trobe University, Melbourne. I chose to examine questions of identity within the framework of the way people with HIV/AIDS construct and manage their lives. The substantive data for the project were drawn from a series of in-depth semistructured interviews with gay men who had HIV/AIDS. I also reflected on my own experience of HIV and situated this in the analysis. Broadly, my inquiry concerned the social construction of identity from the perspective of people with HIV/AIDS. The questions I considered sprang very clearly from my own experience of HIV and my background with HIV/AIDS community organizations. I wanted to trace the processes that contributed to the way the people in my study constructed their identities, and how certain influences, such as interaction with the gay community and the impact of illness, shaped these events.

The study was sociological. In other words, the analysis locates the process of identity construction within broader social parameters where power is exercised and meaning about HIV/AIDS is generated. My aim was to understand these processes from the perspective of the people I interviewed, underpinned by reflections from my experience. The sociological approach was a natural choice because of my background and training as an undergraduate. It was also important to me in other respects.

At the time I started my project much of the social science research on HIV/AIDS was driven by public health policy concerns revolving around transmission and prevention. This is obviously very important work, but it has meant that perspectives situating HIV/AIDS in broader social processes and concerns have been slow to emerge. In addition, research concerned with the experience of HIV/AIDS followed a medical imperative or focused on behavioural issues from the point of view of health professionals. There did not seem to be enough research giving a voice to the broader experiences of people with HIV/AIDS.

I wanted to look at the way in which people with HIV/AIDS managed their identities, as well as understood them. After the extraordinary event of diagnosis, how do people make sense of their changed situation and what are the important influences on their processes of identity change and development? A diagnosis of HIV/AIDS is conferred by medical science, more specifically by the technology of medical science. The diagnosis is, however, meaningful beyond the detection of HIV antibodies. It is the focal point for a contest of meanings involving disease, illness, stigma, death and sex, among other things, and it 'delivers to the individual a new social status' (Arris, 1993).

These seemed to me to be fascinating questions. It is impossible, even reflecting on my motivations for this area of study now, to separate my own desire for personal insight from a more removed intellectual curiosity. The two are inseparable, part of the same thing.

This work was my first major piece of research. The problems I faced as a researcher had as much to do with my inexperience as with my 'insider' status. When I finally settled on my basic research question – how do people with HIV/AIDS manage and construct their identities? – I had to decide on the most suitable approach. Which method and theoretical framework would be the most suitable? Can a person as congenitally chaotic as me possibly hope to manage a project such as this? And a deeper one: am I bright enough to actually pull this off?

INITIAL PROBLEMS

When I was casting around for a research topic I discussed several alternatives, including the one I finally settled on. Right from the start, all the questions I was interested in involved some aspect of HIV/AIDS. It is not surprising to me that I finally decided to address a subject which was the most intimate as far as I was concerned. I had contracted a disease where the issue of identity has a drama and potency approaching that of its physical manifestations. The recent appearance of AIDS, its association with already stigmatized groups, the modes of transmission, the fatal prospect of the disease and the inability of medical science to produce a cure or effective treatment all conspire to make it 'the most political of diseases' (Altman, 1992).

As I write this piece we are over 10 years into the epidemic and, although there have been significant advances in the social position of people with HIV/AIDS, we are still deeply affected by the early social images of the disease. For me, very simply, this means resisting the stigma of the disease at the same time as coping with the possibility of death preceded by a long and painful illness. I need a strong sense of self in order to navigate these issues. Not untypically, I have enjoyed a period of reasonable health since diagnosis. My 'disease career' has so far granted me the time to consider the effect of the HIV on my sense of identity.

There were practical reasons for deciding on this area as well as the desire to satisfy my own curiosity. I had been working with HIV/AIDS community organizations following my diagnosis. When I was thinking about thesis topics I had gained considerable experience of the world of HIV/AIDS community organizations and the broader political framework within which various interests contested and debated the meaning of HIV/AIDS. I knew many people with HIV/AIDS and I was well placed in relation to hearing about changes and developments – medical, social and political. I knew that access to research subjects would not be as difficult for me as for someone who was not known in the area. It seemed to me that if I did not choose to research an area of some familiarity and experience, I would waste much of my knowledge.

Discussions with my supervisor should have been an early warning sign of the problems that I was to face. Initially, although supportive of my decision, he did caution me about the possibility that I would be too close to the work; that the emotional drain of researching an area so intimate to me might cost me dearly. When I told friends about the nature of the research I was involved in, I would sometimes get the sense that they were thinking 'Well that sounds very interesting but why on earth would he want to put himself through that?'

My sense of involvement in the HIV/AIDS community sector seemed to be, at times, almost total. I have spoken to the media as a person with HIV, I have given (and still do from time to time) talks to various groups that involve speaking personally about the experience of HIV. I have worked as a staff member and volunteer for an HIV/AIDS community organization, and I have lost many friends to the disease. It is sometimes very hard to get away from the sense that my entire life is consumed by the issues of AIDS. In my experience this is not an uncommon sensation for people who work in the area. When I started the research for my thesis I was probably at the peak of this involvement. It is the kind of saturation which is all-consuming: very rewarding but also exhausting. The sheer weight of information generated about the disease has meant that at times it has been difficult to retain a perspective that does not personalize everything. In trying to unpack the myriad meanings – personal, social and political – there is a danger of losing a sense of self which is not owed to HIV/AIDS. Concern about the emotional aspect was mirrored by a feeling that my proximity to the issue might produce a piece of work which did not move beyond the familiar contours of the HIV/AIDS discourse.

Through my work I became a part of a collective resistance to the stigmatized construction of HIV/AIDS which has been profoundly influential on the way meaning is created about the disease. This in itself provoked a question about the development of alternative or countervailing identities. They are a necessary prerequisite to the establishment of power in order to challenge the recognized orthodoxies (Altman, 1994). The creation of a powerful identity for people with HIV/AIDS has been an essential condition to establishing a platform from which to negotiate a voice in the HIV/AIDS discourse. In developing an alternative identity through a collective response, however, there is a possibility that, even if stigma is positively reframed, the new identity will impose other regulations and overwhelm individual meaning.

Although my experience grounded me in many of the themes I was to research, I also had to identify and make explicit the ideological content of these themes. I cannot claim that in doing this the work rose above these considerations. AIDS is an intensely political disease riven with ideological interpretations. I can only hope that by making explicit my own position I am able to enter these considerations into the overall framework of the study. The research process meant that I had to question previously taken-for-granted 'facts', and at times this proved uncomfortable. As a researcher engaging in a project from a social constructionist perspective, the implicit questioning of established truth is an ongoing part of the process of research. However, it is one thing to question the truth as represented by powerful institutions such as medicine, but another to bring the critical gaze to bear on groups and political positions that represent your own interests and which you have played a part in establishing. Perhaps the major dilemma for me here was the critical approach I would have to bring to bear on people with HIV/AIDS, their groups and organizations. I have to admit that I was uneasy about this. I do not think that HIV/AIDS organizations and people with HIV/AIDS should be above critical scrutiny, but many such people reside in marginalized pockets of society. They face an enormous task in coping with the daily problems of managing the physical and social aspects of the disease, and I am part of this. It has been said, certainly in relation to HIV/AIDS, that it is easier to criticize if you are a member of the group you are criticizing. The argument behind this runs along the lines that criticism from within cannot be taken as an attempt to disempower or marginalize. Equality of marginalized status guarantees that the criticism is genuine and informed. There may be some truth in this. However, membership of the HIV/AIDS 'club' carries with it complex responsibilities to other people, and one of these is that thoughts and deeds should not add to the already difficult position most people find themselves in.

An example of this is my examination of AIDS activism. Activism seemed to me to embody the paradox of political identity development. In responding to one set of stereotypes it creates another. It is at the same time an important and powerful catalyst for change. AIDS activism offers the tools for people with HIV/AIDS to engage in a dynamic and sometimes dramatic process of identity construction. Activism offers a practical avenue through which to channel power in shaping the political and cultural terrain in which AIDS is played out. More than this though, activism provides people with HIV/AIDS with a concrete focus for the individual construction of meaning around the disease. The influence of activism on identity construction was an interesting and fruitful area of study. My experience working with people with HIV/AIDS had showed me that even if people were not explicitly engaged with an activist organization, they could still feel the power of the activist image. I can only characterize my own career as an activist in lukewarm terms, but my work and my approach to many of the issues of HIV/AIDS has been undeniably influenced by activist considerations. I was conscious of the importance of activism while at the same time maintaining a critique of the effect of activism on identity.

The focus of the study was gay men. Again, the decision to interview only gay men was influenced by my own situation as a person who had participated in the HIV/AIDS self-help community which largely involved gay men, though I am not myself gay. My diagnosis of HIV forced me to look for support – support which at the time was only available from mainly gay groups. My involvement in HIV/AIDS groups has been significant to the way I have managed my own diagnosis and the subsequent events of my life that have been heavily influenced by HIV. Being HIV positive or having AIDS does not necessarily promote a shared sense of identity with others who have the disease. However, certain events and processes which are common to people with HIV do describe the parameters for a commonality of interest, and within these parameters there is ground for the development of identity projects concerned with fashioning a collective response to HIV/AIDS based on the idea of identity, of which I have been a part. In this way, I do consider myself to be a part of a gay community or, more specifically, the community of people with HIV/AIDS within the gay community. However, I am conscious that, although I participated in groups and organizations of people with HIV/AIDS on the basis of my HIV status, and shared in the collective pursuit of the aims and goals of these groups, at the same time I remained somewhat distant because of the underlying gay nature of these groups. What was important in terms of my research is that I approached the work from the perspective of an insider who in some respects was on the outside. The decision to interview gay men, although justified in terms of reducing the variables, owes as much to my curiosity about the relationship between gay identity and the development of HIV/AIDS identity and my own – in my experience – unusual position of being influenced by this.

SITUATING MYSELF IN THE RESEARCH

During my initial thinking about the research I was unclear how I was going to situate myself in the final work. Being the disembodied, disinterested research voice not actively involved, but rather studying and observing, actually quite appealed to me in the early stages of the project. In any case isn't this what science is all about? I do not mean by this that I subscribe to the idea that social science can, by using value-cleansing methods, produce knowledge stripped of all those nasty human qualities like bias and judgement and values; rather, that by engaging in social science research I was aiming for a quality of insight different from that produced by the gaze of the ordinary and everyday. It seems that, despite protestations to the contrary, most researchers, whether qualitative or quantitative, at some level have a residue of the classic scientific ideal. At any rate, the idea of entering the research process explicitly as one of the objects of study was something I resisted. I wanted the work to be somehow above and beyond my own involvement in it. My resistance crumbled, however, when it became apparent that this was not only naive in the extreme but also excluded a valuable set of insights from the research.

I would have had trouble including any of these insights without the acknowledgment that they arose from my own involvement in the area. This being settled, I faced a further problem. How was I to present myself? I went through several options. A personal chapter was the first preferred option. This way I thought that if readers – particularly examiners – did not like this style at least they would only have one chapter of it to endure. However, when I sat down to write it became apparent that, stylistically, as well as in terms of consistency, a discrete first-person account of my experience would look a bit strange beside the rest of the work, where I as an object of the research was not present. I had written much about my experience for conferences and magazines but could not think how I could describe the same things in academic terms. Ultimately, if I wanted the study to reflect my experience and involvement – my insider's knowledge – I had to include myself. The most obvious course was to incorporate my experience into the work where it would have some meaning and make explicit my position in relation to the events I described. That is what I decided to do. It was a process which, at the beginning, made me feel uncomfortably self-conscious. I felt that in some way I was not doing proper research. As I grew more accustomed to the style of writing myself into the study this feeling receded. If my insights as a researcher were valid, why not my experience of HIV/AIDS?

THE INTERVIEWS

Interviews for the study were conducted with six men who were either HIV positive or had AIDS. The interviews were open-ended and lasted from 1½ to 2 hours each. At the outset I had developed a set of core questions to guide the interaction and establish continuity for each interview. The semistructured nature of the interviews allowed the respondents to develop their own themes. This was important. Before the interviews commenced I had only a broad idea of where the study would go. The themes that emerged during the interviews allowed me to refine and focus the analysis. This was also a function of the way the men who were interviewed were recruited. I invited people to take part who I knew had experience of or been exposed to the processes I wanted to investigate.

Interviewing people with HIV/AIDS presents the interviewer with a range of issues to consider. Rose Weitz found that interviewing a group of people with HIV/AIDS presented her with personal, ethical and legal dilemmas (Weitz, 1987). A major concern for Weitz was a responsibility she felt to do justice to the data. Her respondents saw the interview as a legacy they could leave behind to help others. I certainly felt the same responsibility and added a bit of my own. I suppose I was acutely conscious that I did not want to betray the people I was interviewing. This for me was something more than simply doing justice to the data. It was about being a representative of something I shared with the people in my study. Nobody actually said this to me, or even intimated that they knew what kind of finished work they could expect from me. As a researcher I expected that I would produce a piece of work that described and theorized the experiences of the people I interviewed; as an insider I expected the work to be underpinned by the unique insight of someone 'in the know'. These were huge expectations but they seem to me to be inescapable.

The interviews presented me with a number of issues concerned with my own HIV status. About half of the people I interviewed were known to me through community organizations, and I had to be sure that any personal relationship did not bias the data. Checking for inconsistencies was one method of overcoming this. Comparing the transcripts was another.

Another concern was my ability to assume the role of interviewer. The interviews touched on issues very personal to the interviewees: the nature of the information disclosed was intimate and sometimes distressing. I had been involved in similar encounters as part of the work of peer support, an important aspect of which is sharing information and experiences, but during the interviews I was not able to offer this support. I was conscious of this and sometimes I found it difficult to resist the desire to say 'yes, I know that feeling' or talk about my experience when I felt it might be useful. However, once the tape had been turned off and the interview was complete, I saw no reason to impose the same rules.

CONCLUSION

The study is too small to allow me to generalize from the findings. What did emerge, however, is an insight into the issues people face from the pressure generated through the experience of HIV/AIDS. For the individual the challenge is not only to cope with the physical manifestations of the disease but also to make sense of the bewildering array of claims to truth about it; to measure these claims against personal experience, reason and belief, and fashion from this a meaning that can sustain a sense of self against the changes that disease incurs.

From start to finish the research took about 3 years. I do not mean that for those 3 years I devoted myself to my thesis: there were long periods of inactivity punctuated by frenzied activity as guilt got the better of me. My supervisor displayed at times what I thought was an extraordinary amount of patience, for which I was very grateful. When I finally submitted the finished work I was more surprised than relieved. At that time it did occur to me that, throughout the whole process, I was self-imposing a reminder of not only my HIV status but also the potential of illness and death and all the unpleasant baggage that accompanies the disease. However, if I had thought this would be the only outcome I would have chosen another area to research, or just given up. It was at times a very frustrating experience, wondering whether the work I produced was good enough and if I was capable of balancing my role as a researcher with my HIV/AIDS status. I cannot claim that I was able to separate myself from the research. I was intimately involved, the questions I asked of the people I interviewed were questions personal to me. If I had hoped at the outset (which I suspect I did) that in trying to answer these questions through doing research I could distance my personal involvement, or that my role as researcher would somehow shelve my identity as a person with HIV/AIDS, I was mistaken.

On a personal level the research has helped me unravel some of the complex issues that have become a part of my life since diagnosis. As a way of understanding the impact of HIV/AIDS, the research has helped me draw nearer to a clear conception of the intricate social processes involved in the construction of the disease and how I am situated in relation to them. It has not provided me with any blinding personal revelations on how to cope more effectively, nor did I expect it to. But I did acquire important insights into the way people understand and make sense of difficult and traumatic events in their lives. I hope that my research will be of use to others, whether they are people living with HIV/AIDS, researchers working in the area or, like me, a bit of both.

REFERENCES

Altman, D. (1992) The most political of diseases, in *AIDS in Context*, ed E. Timewell, Prentice Hall, Melbourne, pp. 55–72.
Altman, D. (1994) (Homo)sexual identities as a basis for politics, in *Political Identity*, ed G. Stokes, UNSW Press, Sydney, (in press).
Arris, R. (1993) *Against Death: the Sydney Gay Community Responds to AIDS*. PhD Dissertation, Department of Anthropology, Sydney University, New South Wales, Australia.
Homans, G.C. (1970) Contemporary theory in sociology, in *Sociological Methods*, ed N. Denzin, Aldine Publishing Company, Chicago, pp.51–69.
Weitz, R. (1987) The interview as legacy: a social scientist confronts AIDS. *Hastings Center Report* June, 21–3.

CHAPTER 5

Distant voices, still lives: young women, research and (em)power(ment)

Lyn Harrison

My point is not that everything is bad, but that everything is dangerous. (Foucault, 1983, p. 232)
   If one accepts [the]...argument that all data is inherently unstable,
how much is this instability and the otherness of the participants
fully acknowledged in the research report and therefore recognized
as affecting any conclusions? What does it mean to write critically
but less authoritatively when the act of writing is so strongly associated with authority and centrality?

(Opie, 1992, p. 57)

INTRODUCTION

In this chapter (the title of which is a BFI/Film Four production (1988),
director Terence Davies, producer Jennifer Howarth) I want to examine
the notion of 'empowering' research from a feminist poststructuralist perspective using the 'non-directive' conversational interview in qualitative
research as an example. This form of interview is often justified in terms of
its ability to shift power relations by acknowledging and valuing research
participants' voices and experience. This acknowledgement is a recognition that the research participants' experience is as authentic as that of the
researcher. It is argued, however, that this research method mobilizes a
confession discourse which can be both empowering and oppressive. Its
potential for empowerment lies in the discursive spaces it opens up when
voice and experience are valued, and in the pleasure that is generated by
being listened to. However, the discursive practices associated with this
research method can also serve to construct the researcher as knower and

the research participants as 'other' (ignorant, learner, lacking knowledge). The effects of these positionings, however, are never static or predetermined and therefore need to be examined in context.

I will first of all provide background to the study before examining the theoretical problem of power in research relationships. I then provide an illustration and discussion which shows that the valuing of voice and experience is also problematic within what might be termed a general crisis of representation.

BACKGROUND TO THE STUDY

The research reported on here was conducted for my doctoral thesis in health education. The data were collected over a period of 10 months in 1992. The three research participants were young women aged 17 who were in the process of completing their final year at a Victorian secondary school. They were all hoping to commence tertiary education in 1993. All were Anglo-Australian and, at the time this research was conducted, lived in a suburban environment on the outskirts of a large provincial city. I selected these young women because they were normalized as part of mainstream adolescent culture and not radicalized as part of a subcultural group. (Gordon Tait (1993) maintains that distilling particular groups of young people into a subculture transforms and positions individuals into a discrete entity with 'specific codes of behaviour and ways of relating to the outside world'. This does not adequately account for the difference. I would argue that the same holds true for those young people identified as 'normal' who are not labelled as deviant or 'problems' for society and therefore not usually considered worthy research subjects.)

I was concerned to make evident the governing practices that work to construct their 'normal' subjectivities because these practices are so commonplace that they are largely invisible, and are therefore not usually the subject of analysis. This research was guided by a dissatisfaction with media portrayals which consistently failed to capture the complexity of health-related behaviour in the young people I worked with in a variety of contexts. In particular, the representation of young women in such portrayals was, and still is, often defined in relation to masculine norms of youth, adolescence and sexuality, so that the experience of being young and female was either undifferentiated (as if male and female experiences were synonymous) and/or defined as a lack, or was absent altogether.

Initially, the purpose of the research was to find out what 'health' meant to these young women and which health issues were important to them and why. Interviews were conducted fortnightly (with breaks for exams and holidays) during lunchtimes or free periods at school (usually in a 'time-out' room) or in their homes. All interviews were taped and progressively transcribed by me. Copies were sent to the participants before subsequent interviews were scheduled so that we could continually reflect on the data being produced. Because of the level of intensity involved in this type of research I decided that it was necessary to limit the number of participants.

After the first round of interviews I discovered that talking about health resulted in rather stilted question/short answer exchanges. Because my primary methodological concern was to value voice and experience, I decided to discontinue these unsatisfactory conversations and focus the interviews on what these young women wanted to talk about. The interviews therefore became based primarily around their social experiences, both at school and in contexts outside school. Constant reflection on the data produced enabled me to clarify statements made and to pursue particular topics in more depth. The topics canvassed covered a diverse range of subjects, including relationships, pregnancy and motherhood, femininity, the deb ball, schooling and work, and body image. As a result the processes of identity construction emerged as a focus and my research question became 'How is the transition to adulthood constructed by and for young women in relation to their social and bodily health?'

THE 'SUBJECT' OF POSTSTRUCTURALISM

A feminist poststructuralist theory of discourse seemed to offer me a way of connecting these young women's individual experiences to the wider social and cultural processes of identity formation. As Chris Weedon (1993) asserts:

> At the level of the individual, this theory is able to offer an explanation of where our experience comes from, why it is contradictory or incoherent and why and how it can change.

Because poststructuralism offers a theory of the relation between language, subjectivity, social organization and power (Weedon, 1988) it is attractive to feminists, who have a common interest in uncovering the ways in which women are systematically oppressed as well as in how 'gender power relations are constituted, reproduced and contested' (Weedon, 1988).

Like all theories, poststructuralism promotes a particular view of the world that cannot and does not pretend to be compatible with all feminist discourses and political agendas. But, as Weedon maintains, it does offer 'a useful, productive framework for understanding the mechanisms of power in our society and the possibilities of change'.

From a feminist poststructuralist perspective people are seen as agentic subjects who are able to make choices '...within a range of socially available discursive positions, molding and creatively adapting discourses as they act' (Leahy, 1994; see also Davies, 1989; Smith, 1988; Weedon, 1988).

Poststructuralist approaches offer a concept of agency that is limited by the subject positions made available in discourse. Nevertheless, subjects can and do 'choose positions between discourses, choose from a variety of subject positions within a particular discourse, or create new subject positions' (Leahy, 1994; see also Alcoff, 1988).

Discourse, in the context in which it is used here, refers to '...a socially constructed set of statements – a linked set of terms, interpretations, meanings, evaluations and causal analyses' (Leahy, 1994). Although the relationship between discourse and social practice is not one of causality, social practices are a part of the discursive field; they are '...situated within and enunciate specific discourses' (Leahy, 1994) and as such 'every practice is by definition both discursive and material (Henriques *et al.*, 1984). Discourses do not set out what is true or false but '...what can have a truth-value...or in other words, what is statable' and thinkable and therefore what is desirable. They work through 'systems of exclusion such as the prohibition of certain words, the division between mad and sane speech, and the (historically contingent) disjunction between true and false' (Alcoff and Gray, 1993). More than one discourse can circulate in any given context and these discourses exist in a hierarchical relationship to one another. As Foucault (1978) states:

> Discourse transmits and produces power, it reinforces it, but also undermines and exposes it, renders it fragile and makes it possible to thwart it.

In this formulation the world is not divided neatly between dominant and dominated discourses. Discourses are inherently unstable and it is only by studying their effects in practice that their liberatory status can be determined. Keenan (1987, cited in Gore, 1993) argues that 'because the articulation between power and knowledge is discursive, then the link can never be guaranteed'. Some feminists have found Foucault's discourse theory useful because it offers a non-deterministic approach to power and an understanding of positionality which allows for the possibility of change. (Linking Foucault with feminism is not unproblematic: see McNay (1992) and Sawicki (1991), both of whom provide a detailed analysis of the positive and negative aspects of such a partnership.)

The concept of positionality is integral to poststructuralist formulations of the subject. When we think or speak we position ourselves within a field of particular historically (re)produced discourses. Our identity is not just the product of external social and cultural relations. Nor is it innate, or somehow external to these relations, as essentialist formulations of identity would have us believe (women are 'naturally' nurturing). Instead, our identity 'is the product of [our]... own interpretation and reconstruction of [our]... history, as mediated through the cultural context to which [we]... have access' (Alcoff, 1988).

In seeking to explain why people take up subject positions in one dis-course rather than another, Hollway (1984) points to the need to pay attention to the histories of individuals '...in order to see the recursive positioning in certain positions in discourse' as well as the investment individuals have in taking up these positions. Outlining what she means by investment, Hollway states:

> By claiming that people have investments ...in taking up certain positions in discourses, and consequently in relation to each other, I mean that there will be some satisfaction or pay-off or reward ...for that person. The satisfaction may well be in contradiction with other resultant feelings. It is not necessarily conscious or rational. But there is a reason.

Hollway theorizes the reason for investment in terms of power and the way it historically constructs individual subjectivity. Recursive positioning in frequently used discourses gives us a coherent sense of self and because of this we have a strong investment in maintaining particular subject posi-tions (Davies, 1991).

EMPOWERMENT

The valuing of voice and experience in feminist research is potentially dangerous if these categories are viewed as self-evident and not socially constructed and culturally mediated within a network of power relations.

Feminist research is often framed as essentially liberating, democratic, emancipatory, empowering and able to value and encourage women's 'voice'. It is sometimes these things but it is equally true to say that some-times it is undemocratic, oppressive and silencing. The effects of dis-courses can only be determined within particular contexts. Further, 'issues of trust, risk, and the operations of fear and desire around such issues of identity and politics' (Ellsworth, 1989) need to be addressed because '...knowledge, power and desire are mutually implicated' (Ellsworth, 1989; see also Henriques *et al.*, 1984) in the constitution of our sense of self, and necessarily guide our practices.

Ellsworth describes empowerment, (student) voice and dialogue as they are framed within critical pedagogy as '...repressive myths that per-petuate relations of domination'. To support her argument she asserts that the same categories within feminist pedagogy have different effects because these metaphors '...are conceptualized in terms of 'self-defini-tions' that are oppositional to definitions of women constructed by oth-ers'. This was one of the taken-for-granted assumptions that informed the research project reported on here. Self-definitions in this context are taken to be somehow more authentic than other definitions. Ellsworth is careful elsewhere to emphasize how she and her students are multiply positioned along the lines of class, age, gender, ableness, race, ethnicity etc. She cites Trinh Minh-ha to support this proposition:

> There are no social positions exempt from becoming oppressive to others...any group – any position – can move into the oppressor role. (Trinh. T. Minh-ha, 1986/87, cited in Ellsworth, 1989).

It follows, then, that feminist discourses cannot somehow exist outside relations of power and, despite intentions to the contrary, they do have the potential to be as oppressive as other discourses.

POWER – KNOWLEDGE

Gore (1993) suggests that so-called liberatory pedagogies have their own 'regimes of truth' which are 'the ensemble of rules according to which the true and the false are separated and specific effects of power attached to the true' (Foucault, 1980). Gore understands regime of truth as '...the connection between power and knowledge which is produced by, and produces, a specific act of government'.

Gore states that both feminist and critical pedagogies are framed within a 'modernist construction of power' which sees power as domination, or, as she frames it, 'repressive power' and 'power as the property of some over others'. More disconcertingly, she states that '...such a notion of power is necessary if the idea of empowerment is to be plausible'. In this formulation the notion of empowerment carries with it an agent of empowerment (someone, or something, doing the empowering), a notion of power as property (to empower implies to give or confer power) and a vision or desired end state (some vision of what it is to be empowered and the possibility of a state of empowerment). This notion of empowerment is problematic because it tends to take on a totalizing logic when it is viewed in terms of either/or, empowering/dizempowering (Gore, 1993).

Explicit in the notion of empowerment is the view that students' understandings of their lived experience are somehow incomplete or lacking and need to be brought up '...to the teacher's level of understanding' (Ellsworth, 1989). This notion of empowerment presumes they [students or research participants] need other knowledges or in fact want them; that they cannot work this out for themselves or, even if they can, that they will welcome being brought into the light (Ellsworth, 1989). Ellsworth also points out that this formulation fails to acknowledge the teacher's 'partial' knowledge, history, values etc. which make problematic the idea that the teacher [or researcher] can 'bring subjugated knowledges to light' when we are 'not free of [our]...own learned racism, fat oppression, classism, ableism, or sexism'.

Furthermore, institutional structures set up a hierarchical relationship between teacher knowledge and student knowledge that strategies such as student empowerment and dialogue fail to dismantle. Ellsworth acknowledged this when she stated that her institutional role 'would always weight [her] statements differently from those of students'. Those who engage in liberatory research projects need to examine their own implication in the production of regimes of truth. Our own partial knowledge is brought to the fore by the act of engaging with others and reflecting on that engagement, and it then becomes evident that our multiple strands of identity are worked through differently at different times and in different places.

EXPERIENCE

An acknowledgement of the partiality of experience means that researchers can no longer position themselves as the disinterested mediators on the side of the 'oppressed' group. Ellsworth has made the point that she 'could not unproblematically 'affiliate' with the social groups [her]...students represented and interpret their experience to them' (Ellsworth, 1989). This was also the case in my research. Although I found echoes of myself in the experiences these young women related to me, for me they were of another time and another place and I was looking at them through eyes that had seen, and a body that had experienced, at least 20 years more than theirs had. Ellsworth urges us as teachers and researchers to acknowledge that we are always implicated in the very structures we are trying to change, and that when we affiliate with other social groups in an effort to try and interpret their experience to them we are engaging in practices that are in danger of stripping their speech of authority and authenticity.

In my everyday experiences (as is the case with everyone) my positioning constructs, and is constructed through, my own history and social and cultural hierarchies of knowledge/taste/morals/preconceptions/suppositions. I have 'standards' (not always rational, nor set in concrete) which are guides to action/behaviour/thoughts. I cannot shrug them off in the social process of doing research. This does not mean that I am unable to interpret and analyse the experiences of others, but it does mean that these interpretations will always be partial.

Basing research around the experiences of marginalized groups (in this context young women) is often seen as an important corrective to traditional dominant 'constructions of social worlds' because it uncovers a 'world of alternative values and practices' (Scott, 1991) which challenge these constructions. Although Scott is referring explicitly here to the writing of histories that call on authentic experience to support claims to truth, her insights are applicable to all areas of the social sciences concerned with the politics of difference. Scott emphasizes the importance of social accounts that document the lives of those previously omitted or overlooked in 'conventional histories'. However, she wishes to make problematic the notion of experience as a 'reflection of the real'. Michel deCertau (cited in Scott, 1991) maintains that historical discourse is made credible by its supposed representation of 'reality' but that 'this authorized appearance of the 'real' serves precisely to camouflage the practice which in fact determines it'. As Scott asks, '...what could be truer, after all, than a subject's account of what he or she has lived through?' Her concern here is that by casting experience as an 'originary point of explanation' the critical thrust of 'histories of difference' is weakened. The danger here is that:

> Questions about the constructed nature of experience, about how subjects are constituted as different in the first place, about how one's vision is structured – about language (or discourse) and history – are left aside. The evidence of experience becomes evidence for the fact of difference, rather than a way of exploring how difference is established, how it operates, how and in what ways it constitutes subjects, who see and act in the world. (Scott, 1991)

By calling on the evidence of 'authentic' experience, therefore, difference is naturalized and the stories of marginalized others become just another way of being in the world. Such a view disguises the fact that 'difference is relationally constituted' (Scott, 1991), that is, we are only different in relation to others. As Scott points out, we need to go further and attend to the 'historical processes that, through discourse, position subjects and produce experiences'. This is not to deny subjective experience since, as Chris Weedon points out, '...the ways in which people make sense of their lives is a necessary starting point for understanding how power relations structure society'. However, any account of experience needs to be able to show '...where it comes from and how it relates to material social practices and the power relations which structure them'.

Alcoff and Gray (1993) assert that the production of personal narratives can essentialize experience and identity if these narratives are presented as 'simple reports, thus obscuring the way in which all experience is discursively mediated'. In this context Bell Hooks (1989) believes that it is 'necessary to move beyond simply naming experience to placing that experience in a theoretical context' in order to make personal experience politically useful and transformative.

VOICE

> Speech is an event involving an arrangement of speakers and hearers; it is an act in which relations get constituted and experience and subjectivities are mediated. (Alcoff and Gray, 1993)

Before judgements can be made about speaking out as a form of empowerment it is necessary to take account of the context of speaking:

who speaks, who does not speak, when and why, what position they speak from, as well as the effects of such speaking. This context is important because any speaking out is 'predicated on the absence and marginalization of alternative voices' and 'is the result of conscious and unconscious assessments of the power relations and safety of the situation' (Ellsworth, 1989).

Should we be speaking for others?

All acts of speaking, whether speaking to, for, about or with (this includes doing and writing research as a form of all of these), are political acts. Not speaking also has political consequences. Alcoff (1991) addresses some of the issues identified in contemporary debates which are concerned about the possibility or even the desirability of speaking for others. She points out that where we speak from is important because 'certain privileged locations are discursively dangerous'. As academics, for example, we are authorized, by virtue of our position in the academy, to theorize the 'ideas, needs, and goals of others'. Alcoff urges us to start questioning whether this is a legitimate authority. Trinh Minh-ha (cited in Alcoff, 1991) has some strong opinions on this subject:

'Them' always stands on the other side of the hill, naked and speechless...'them' is only admitted among 'us', the discussing subjects, when accompanied or introduced by an 'us'.

Minh-ha points to the potential for all research to colonize those being researched and to turn them into exotic 'others'.

Some see a solution in only speaking for groups of which we are a member, but this stance is problematic because we are all multiply positioned along lines of race, class, gender, age, ethnicity and so on. Alcoff poses the question 'Can a white woman speak for all women simply by virtue of being a woman?' and 'If not, how narrowly should we draw the categories?' Hooks chooses to speak and write from a black woman's perspective. This is a political stance which seeks to disrupt the generic category 'woman' but may have the effect of eliding 'differences' among black women. Alcoff does not offer answers to the questions she poses but instead points to the fact that if you restrict speaking for others to groups of which you are a member this is not in itself an easy solution. But what of those who speak for others who are not members of their own social and /or cultural group? Alcoff acknowledges that all speakers lose a portion of control over the meaning and truth of their utterances because they can never know everything about the context of their speech, and with electronic communication it is 'difficult to know anything at all about the context of reception' (Alcoff, 1991). However, she does not see this as an excuse for abdicating responsibility or refusing to be accountable for what we write and say.

Deciding to resolve this problem by only speaking for yourself is also problematic. Speaking only for yourself can be viewed as a retreat from responsibility and accountability, and actually assumes a level of autonomy from others that does not exist (Alcoff, 1991). Even if you retreat from speaking for others and maintain that you are only speaking for yourself you are still representing yourself in a particular way. As Alcoff states: '...I am constructing a possible self...and am offering that to others...as one possible way to be'. Addressing another dimension of the same problem, Spivak (cited in Alcoff, 1991) takes issue with what she describes as the 'self-abnegating intellectual' (she has Foucault, among others, in mind here) because this retreat position assumes that '...the oppressed can transparently represent their own interests' as if experience were 'transparent and self-knowing' which essentializes the oppressed as 'non-ideologically constructed subjects'. Even a complete retreat from speaking at all is a political act because it allows the 'continued dominance of current discourses' (Alcoff, 1991).

So, what are we to do if speaking to, for, with, about or indeed not at all are all potentially dangerous? Alcoff points out that the problem of speaking for others 'exists in the very structure of discursive practice' and that it is this 'structure that needs alteration' (Alcoff, 1991). She also points out that developing alternatives requires a great deal of theoretical and practical work, and that until then 'the practice of speaking for others remains the best possibility in some existing situations'. This is not in itself a retreat position, but an acknowledgement that we do not have all the answers. As is the case with any speaking out (no matter what the problems), Alcoff's speaking out has the potential to subvert and challenge existing power relations and knowledge production. Being aware of the dangers can help us to lessen them. One way of doing this is to deconstruct our own practice in an attempt to uncover particular power relations and their discursive effect. Moreover, as Alcoff says:

> It is not always the case that when others unlike me speak for me I have ended up worse off, or that when we speak for others they end up worse off. Sometimes, as Loyce Stewart has argued, we do need a 'messenger' to advocate for our needs. (Alcoff, 1991)

In the context of this research I am acting as a 'messenger' to advocate for the needs of Kate, Nadine and Sara (the pseudonyms chosen by the three young women in this project). At the same time I am aware of the dangers of taking on such a position.

ON RESEARCH AS CONFESSION

We need new ways to analyze the personal and the political as well as new ways to conceptualize these terms. Experience is not 'pretheoretical', nor is theory separate or separable from experience, and both are always already political. A project of social change, therefore, does not need to 'get beyond' the personal narrative or the confessional to become political but rather needs to analyze the various effects of the confessional in different contexts and to create discursive spaces in which we can maximize its disruptive effects. (Alcoff and Gray, 1993)

The non-directive interview is closely related to the confession in both its discursive practice and its aims and, as Oakley (1981) points out, is derived directly from the language of psychotherapy, a field in which the confession finds its secular genesis.

McHoul and Grace cite several forms of the confession: interviews, conversations and autobiographical narratives among them. The point they make is that no matter what form the confession takes it is a 'ritual which unfolds within a power relationship'. As Foucault (1978) has stated:

...the confession became one of the West's most highly valued techniques for producing truth. We have since become a singularly confessing society. The confession has spread its effects far and wide. It plays a part in justice, medicine, education, family relationships, and love relations, in the most ordinary affairs of everyday life, and in the most solemn rites; one confesses one's crimes, one's sins, one's thoughts and desires, one's illnesses and troubles; one goes about telling, with the greatest precision, whatever is most difficult to tell. One confesses in public and in private, to one's parents, one's educators, one's doctor, to those one loves; one admits to oneself, in pleasure and in pain, things it would be impossible to tell to anyone else, the things people write books about... Western man [sic] has become a confessing animal.

Even though Foucault suggests that the confession is an instrument of domination it is also 'an important site of struggle in which domination and resistance are played out' (Alcoff and Gray, 1993).

Alcoff and Gray point out that those confessing disclose their 'innermost experiences to an expert mediator who then reinterprets those experiences back to her using the dominant discourse's codes of normality'. In the context in which they are writing (related to the discourse of those who have survived rape, incest and sexual assault) Alcoff and Gray maintain that those who speak out are 'inscribed in dominant structures of subjectivity; their own subjectivities being increasingly subsumed under hegemonic discourse'. Although in the context of my discussions with the three young women participating in my research study feminist discourse can hardly be described in these terms, it still has the potential for subsuming the subjectivities of these young women.

Weedon (1987) maintains that 'to speak is to assume a subject position within discourse and to become subjected to the power and regulation of discourse'. Within the confessional mode of the non-directive interview the subject positions available are limited (although not incapable of being changed or expanded). My position as researcher/interviewer invests me with the authority to ask questions, to solicit and pass judgement on the confession (Weedon, 1987). This has the effect of stripping those who confess of authority and agency (Alcoff and Gray, 1993). Those being interviewed are positioned as 'the speaking subject'. This positioning has multiple and contradictory effects which can be empowering and oppressive at the same time. These young women's positioning as speaking subjects within the research discourse cannot be divorced from their discursive production as young, female and student, in which they are, more often than not, also stripped of authority or agency. Here 'student' agency is a complex phenomenon because the effective teacher/student relationship relies not just on compliance but on the agentic good will of the student. Similarly, my discursive production as researcher cannot be divorced from my positioning as adult. Although we are all female and students, age and differential institutional positioning and histories mediate experience here so that my statements are weighted differently from those of the young women (Ellsworth, 1989). This is particularly so when it comes to writing up the research (this chapter is an example).

How do these different discursive positions work to structure the network of power relations in the context of this research? More often than not, being a young student means not speaking. The old adage 'children should be seen but not heard' is appropriate here. When students speak out in the classroom environment or in other relationships with adults/teachers they risk admonishment. If they ask questions they can draw attention to themselves, risking embarrassment by acknowledging that they do not understand something. As one of the research participants stated:

> It's very hard especially if you are embarrassed if it's something simple. You know like it may not be something that you have learned but everyone else seems to know what they're doing...(Kate, 26/6/92).

It should be emphasized that asking questions is not always seen as difficult or embarrassing and the degree of difficulty seems to be dependent on particular teachers, the sort of question you want to ask, and the level of confidence that each student has in her abilities over a range of subjects. If you are positioned as a 'good' student, asking questions is part of your discursive practice. The quality of face-to-face relations also seems to be an important mitigating factor here. Generally speaking, however, if the type of questions asked makes it obvious that you do not understand something then the risk of exposing your ignorance to others and the wish not to seem too interested in school work (present in various degrees in each of the participants) means that asking questions is often seen as a risky undertaking. Here the role of teachers as transmitters of knowledge, invested with the power to ask questions of students, is similar to my discursive production as a researcher. Although the quality of face-to-face relationships in the research context may well have been different from that of teacher/student interaction, this positioning authorizes me to ask questions and to make affirming statements, which encourages them to talk about their experiences (Alcoff and Gray, 1993).

One of the dangers of the confessional mode of research is that participants' speech transformed into data becomes a commodity (Alcoff and Gray, 1993). Its value lies in the ability of the researcher to integrate participants' speech by interpretation and a suitable theoretical framework, into a piece of academic writing (in this case a thesis), which is then judged on its originality or extension of knowledge in the field in which it is situated. This after all is the aim of this type of research. Its consequence, however, is that I am not subject to the same imperative to self-disclose as are the young women. (Extra)ordinary experiences and voices are thus transformed – doubly mediated as data and then as thesis – ghosts with shadowy bodies and voices that only faintly echo.

Alcoff and Gray (1993), writing about how 'survivor discourse' has become a media event on American talkback television programmes such as 'Donahue', state that the value of survivor speech is based on its sensationalism and drama. Although the production of a thesis is not subject to the same imperatives, decisions about what data are included and what are not are often made for reasons that are not always guided by a concern for what may be the best interests of participants. The common practice of using pseudonyms, for instance, presupposes the dangers of self-disclosure that are not inherent in survey-type research.

Related to this, the discursive structure of the confessional works to establish a binary opposition between empirical experience and theory. As Alcoff and Gray (1993) point out:

> The confessional mode also reproduces the notion of 'raw experience' and sets up binary structures between experience and theory, feelings and knowledge, subjective and objective, and mind and body. These binaries are instantiated in the discursive arrangement of the confessional, which splits speaking roles on the basis of these divisions. Such a split is not only possible but considered necessary for the development of a credible theory because of the internal structure of the binary, which subordinates one term to the other. The first part of the binary – experience, feelings, emotional pain – provides the raw data needed to produce theory and knowledge.

Raw experience here is privileged over, and necessary for, the production of theory in its role as 'objective assessment' and academic knowledge production. But there other binaries working here, such as adult/young person, which complicate as they work to reinforce the split between experience and theory. Whose experience holds? The interpreter, as I have suggested above, is the more powerful within the adult/young person binary.

However, these binaries are not immutable. If we acknowledge that the discursive practice of research mobilizes these binary oppositions, then naming and writing about them are important steps if we are to imagine how they might be otherwise. It is also the case that we all experience the effects of these binary oppositions (no matter which side of the divide we are positioned on) in different ways, depending on our different social and cultural locations and differential histories. I will return to this point later.

For the research participants 'feeling safe to speak' is a desirable prerequisite in the context of the interview, but it cannot be abstracted from what the researcher does with this speaking.

INTERVIEWING YOUNG WOMEN: SPEAKING TO, WITH, FOR AND AGAINST

Speaking with friends

Sharpe (1994) has suggested that 'the importance of friends for many teenagers at this time in life cannot be underestimated' as they act as important reference points in young people's search for meaning and identity. In the context of this research it was evident that speaking with friends was integral to peer relationship maintenance for Kate, Nadine and Sara. These young women would gather in the lunchroom or at their favourite sites in the school grounds and gossip about boys, upcoming or past social events, problems they had with parents or teachers, or the latest development in their favourite soaps. They would 'hit' the telephone as soon as they walked in the door at home to talk with their friends about homework, or things that happened at school that they had not had time to reflect on or discuss during the day, or problems with boyfriends. Talk among peers was an affirming practice. They were able to voice their concerns and insecurities in an environment that was, for the most part, non-judgemental. Talking is an important connecting practice in the process of identity construction for young women. Labelling their talk as gossip often devalues its importance as a form of relationship maintenance and identity construction.

Speaking to adults

Although talking with friends is self-affirming the same cannot be said about young people talking with adults. Apart from parent/daughter exchanges the young women in this research talked mainly about teacher/student relationships. Teachers are the main source of adult contact that these young women experience outside the family. Leaving aside the quality of relationships between different teachers, teachers still exist as authority figures and interactions are primarily based around the teacher as knower and the student as receiver of knowledge. This means that student voices are invariably heard in relation to school knowledge. When other knowledges or experiences surface they are judged on their relationship with, and adaptability to, school knowledge. Of course, for those whose patterns of interaction and knowledge acquisition closely resemble those present in the school setting, this is less of a problem.

On the positive side research that seeks to value a whole range of knowledge and experiences outside the school setting does open up the possibility for these young women to interact with adults in a different way, which at the very least has the potential to be empowering. However, as is the case with any relations of power the effects cannot be predicted. Seeking to value voice and experience does not automatically lead to empowerment. Weedon (1987) states that 'Those interests which a discourse serves may be far from which it appears, at first sight, to represent'. One of the dangers of this type of research is that it makes these young women's experiences public in a much broader sense than they would normally be, and therefore open to scrutiny and analysis by academics such as myself. This may actually provide another form of surveillance of the young by adults (Foucault, 1977).

The discursive practices of the confessional mean that the confessor is not just 'the other party to the dialogue' (Weedon, 1987) 'but the authority who requires the confession, prescribes and appreciates it, and intervenes in order to judge, punish, forgive, console and reconcile' (Foucault, 1978).

Although it is necessary to examine power relations in particular contexts between particular individuals in order not to overdetermine the discursive positions made available in confessional discourse (a point I will return to shortly), Foucault has pointed to the power structure immanent in the confession discourse, which means that the interviewer as confessor is not subject to the same imperatives to speak and self-disclose as the subject who confesses (Foucault, 1978).

As a counter to this position Oakley (1981) argues that in the interview situation the women she studied frequently asked questions which challenged the question-asking and rapport-promoting role of the interviewer, and the view of interviewees as passive. After rereading Oakley (1981) I decided to revisit my data and document the type and the frequency of questions asked by the participants. I initially used the four categories of questions Oakley used in her analysis. She defined her types of questions as personal (questions about her attitudes or experiences); questions about the research (Are you going to write a book?); advice questions (Do you think...? How long do I...?); and information requests (who will deliver my baby?). However, I found that I needed to add another category, which I named 'clarifying questions' to account for questions that did not easily conform to any of Oakley's four categories (Our age you mean? Who? The guys or..?). This categorization and the breakdown and frequency of questioning of each participant is presented in Table 5.1.

Table 5.1 Questions interviewees asked

Type of question	Kate	Sara	Nadine
Personal	33	1	1
Clarification	18	10	18
Research	20	–	1
Advice	2	–	–
Information	14	15	20
Total	87	26	40

Oakley's research was on the transition to motherhood and her interviewees' information requests covered medical procedures, organizational procedures, physiology or reproduction, and baby care/development/feeding and other (unspecified). In the context of my research the information requests were much more far-ranging, considering we canvassed topics initiated by the young women that covered areas as diverse as schoolwork, the deb ball, diet, teenage pregnancy, boyfriends, family – the list goes on. What is significant for my analysis is the discrepancy between Kate and the other two young women in regard to personal questions and questions about the research. This is not easily explained by differential positioning within the confession discourse as, on the surface at least, our researcher/subject relationships were identical. Why was it that Kate asked so many more personal questions and questions about the research than either Sara or Nadine?

From a poststructuralist perspective we would need to try and uncover what other discursive positions interact with or contradict the positions available in the confession discourse. The concept of investment (Hollway, 1984) I outlined earlier is useful here. As always, my observations are based on my always partial knowledge of the different subject positions made available to these young women. These are not self-evident in the interview transcripts and my observations and analysis rely in no small part on interactions that were neither taped nor transcribed. In the case of Kate and Nadine I have a history of working with them on youth projects not connected with this research over a period of 3 years. My acquaintanceship with Sara was in the context of this research only. Interactions with people in different contexts can be helpful in determining what other discourses might affect the power relations evident in any one particular context. However, these intentions are not always helpful in changing these power relations, because to a certain extent the problem exists in the very structure of discursive practice itself (Alcoff, 1991).

To help investigate this problem I will now consider my research relationships with each of the young women, using as illustration both a particular exchange between one of the young women in this research and myself and more holistic accounts of the research relationship with the others.

KATE

Kate and I had been talking about her recent decision to join Weight Watchers. Her diet was very similar to the diabetic diet that I follow and I commented on this to her. She then said:

Kate: I never knew you were a diabetic.

L: Didn't you?

Kate: You're full of secrets. Last week I found out you smoke and this week I find out you are a diabetic.

L: The thing is I always ask you the questions and you never ask me, so you should ask (laughing).

K: I'm not going to ask 'Are you a diabetic?' (Interview, 11/9/92)

Kate's use of the word 'secrets' is significant here. I did not consciously set out to keep secrets but I was consciously, explicitly, positioned here by Kate as having them. The confessional discourse that was mobilised for this research positioned Kate as 'speaker' and 'knower', and until this point (which was quite late in the research process) this was the pattern of interaction. As I noted above, however, positioning in particular discourses is not immutable, and after this exchange Kate asked a lot more questions related both to my own personal circumstances and to the research we were engaged in. She asked me to confess my secrets, in effect. Here, Kate was able to reverse and appropriate the subject positions available in the confession discourse and position me as confessing. This was not the case with the other two young women who participated in the research.

Although asking more questions of me changed our relationship the effects were not always positive. All of the young women knew each other. They were in the same year at the same school and Sara and Kate were part of the same friendship group. Both Kate and Nadine were members of the same youth network; it was via my work with this group that I came to know Nadine and Kate in the first place. Nadine, however, was not a friend of either Sara or Kate and she did not refer to either of them in the context of our interviews. Sara did not refer to Nadine, although she did refer to Kate. Likewise Kate referred to Sara but not to Nadine; not, that is, until after the interview I have reported here. Shortly after this critical incident with Kate, Nadine found out that she was pregnant. My changed research relationship with Kate enabled her to start asking questions about Nadine's pregnancy and her reaction to it, questions that I interpreted as gossip. Although Nadine's pregnancy could have been expected to generate gossip amongst her peers it had been an unspoken rule that our interviews were not the forum for such discussions. This placed me in a difficult position as far as confidentiality was concerned: I did not want to encourage Kate to talk about the other participants, nor did I want to return to a position where I asked all the questions and she answered them. Talking about Nadine only reinforced the transgressive nature of her pregnancy in terms of her positioning as a 'young (too young to be pregnant) student'. As a result my answers were non-commital and I quickly sought to change the subject.

NADINE

Nadine, in the contexts in which I knew her, always positioned herself as knower, as independent, as in charge and capable of bucking the system. In other contexts she always asked questions and was forceful in her opinions. In the context of my research she also positioned herself as knower and as independent. What she did not do, however, was ask questions related to the research. Nor did she ask personal questions. Here the notion of investment is important. Nadine, more than the other two young women, was keen to use the research as a tool: as a means of maintaining a research profile that had the potential to help her in future pursuits outside the context of schooling. This is a perfectly legitimate reason for participating in the research and is potentially more empowering than research participation based around altruistic reasons. If participants have an idea that there will be a pay-off for their participation it seems more likely that they will set themselves limits about their level of commitment. This meant that Nadine might not have been interested in what motivated me to do this type of research, or in what the research might uncover.

Nadine was the only one who failed to turn up for prearranged interviews without notifying me; she was the only one who yawned when she answered the door to me; she ate and rattled lolly papers during recording, or played with her dog or suddenly stopped in mid-sentence to talk with her mother. She had other friends around when we were interviewing and interviews were often conducted with her in a supine position on the couch, or moving about the room. She was the only one who indicated explicitly that her time was limited and that she always had other things to do. Although none of these practices broke the confession cycle they served to remind me that the interviews were to be conducted on her terms. These practices cannot be read from the interview transcripts, which highlights the limitations of only attending to what people say through the disembodied analysis of words on a page.

The quality of face-to-face relations is an important research consideration because, as Evelyn Fox Keller says, '...data never do speak for themselves' (1985, cited in Lenzo, 1994). When these relations are characterized by ambivalence, or sometimes antagonism, it makes it more difficult to attend to and value what people say.

SARA

I would now like to turn to my relationship with Sara, who thus far has been an absent presence. Sara was a 'good' student. She was hardworking, conscientious, keen to succeed and eager to please. She came into the research only after another young woman withdrew from the project due to other commitments. In our interactions she was initially much quieter and more hesitant in expressing herself. Although this changed as the research progressed our relationship was always much more formal than my relationship with Kate and Nadine. It more closely resembled the interaction between teacher and student, and because this interaction is closely related to the discursive practice of the confession Sara was also a 'good' research participant. When I asked her to write something for me it was always ready. She always worked hard to accommodate my schedule and always rang me well ahead if she had to cancel.

In Sara's case the formal boundaries placed around the research worked as a form of resistance to self-disclosure. This resistance was most evident whenever the subject of teenage sexuality was broached by me. With all three young women I used two newspaper surveys on adolescent sexuality as an impetus for discussions at different stages in the research. During these discussions with Sara I always felt that I was crossing her implicitly pre-existing boundary of acceptable researcher/researched relations.

It was not that Sara did not answer my questions or offer opinions but she stuck very closely to talking about the articles, avoiding any personal revelations. She did not seek to extend discussions as the other young women did. With Kate and Nadine we discussed such things as personal condom use, gender relations, and cultural expectations and stereotypes. Although Sara and I did discuss gender relations, cultural expectations and stereotypes I was unable to generate the same level of engagement with her as I had with Kate and Nadine. This does not imply any hierarchical value judgements about the information gained from these interviews. Instead, it points to the different discourses that these young women were positioned in and the different knowledges produced in these discourses. In my position as confessor I could have pushed the point and asked harder questions. However, my concern to be a caring researcher, not to conduct research that was overly intrusive, and to be guided by what the young women wanted to talk about prevented me from doing this. With all that is written about adolescent sexuality and the endless surveys that this topic seems to generate one might be forgiven for thinking that sex and sexuality were pre-eminent in the hearts and minds of the young, and more importantly that they feel comfortable talking to strangers about their sexuality.

Sara herself, when talking about the newspaper surveys I showed her, commented that it is much easier to tick a box where there is little or no accountability for the answers you give and you remain anonymous:

> I'd say it must...it would have to be a survey with just ticking boxes...cos it wouldn't because they wouldn't ask you to sort of describe every detail cos otherwise they wouldn't get all these people...it would have to be an easy tick the box thing...yes/no. (Interview, 21/12/92)

Later Sara speculated on the possibility that it is easy to exaggerate or lie about your sexual habits in a 'tick the box' survey. It is much harder to talk about such issues face to face with someone over a lengthy period of time, knowing that the person you confess to intends to examine and analyse everything you say. This was not something that appeared to concern Nadine or Kate, but there may well be a price to be paid for their self-disclosure. Both Nadine and Kate have a chapter in my thesis devoted to each of them. Sara, on the other hand, appears mainly in another chapter where all three young women are given almost equal space. As a consequence my portrayals of Nadine and Kate are clearly much more dangerous in the sense that their experiences are made open to public scrutiny in ways that Sara's are not. Related to this, Ellsworth (1989) states that:

> ...the assumption present in the literature that silence in front of a teacher or professor indicates 'lost voice', 'voicelessness' or lack of social identity from which to act as a social agent betrays deep and unacceptable gender, race, and class [and age] biases.

In the context of my research encouraging young women to 'speak out' presupposes that they will actually benefit from talking about their experiences. Although in some instances self-scrutiny may be beneficial, as I have mentioned previously, it also has the potential to be threatening and destabilizing (Taylor, 1993). Ellsworth (1989) points out that students' speaking out involves a complex form of strategizing on their part 'for the visibility that speech gives without giving up the safety of silence'. Sara, for instance, using a form of agency available to her as a good student to comply but not engage, retains this agency and/or expresses this strategizing, which has the effect of making her less vulnerable to scrutiny. The others also act agentically but in a different way, with different outcomes. Kate, by engaging more (too much?), certainly changes the rules of the interview but this makes her more vulnerable.

CONCLUSION

Research with young people in education and in the social and health sciences has a long tradition of using qualitative methods to study so-called deviant or subcultural groups (Willis, 1977; Roman, 1987; Walker, 1988; McLaren, 1989) and relies on a privileging of experience collected as data, and as a means of generating valid theory. My intention was to move away from identifying a particular subcultural group to study because I did not want to reinforce and construct any particular group as deviant, or position them as exotic others. I decided not to engage in participant observation because of this concern. I now realize that my choice of research participants and methods was based around some problematic assumptions. The first assumption was that research on subcultural groups was first and foremost an act of violence, with little or no benefit accruing to members of the group/s being researched. This view serves to deny members of such groups agency and a capacity for co-optation or resistance. Secondly, and this is related to the first point, I assumed that it was possible to do research with real people (as opposed to texts) that was not a form of violence as long as you chose the right methods (feminist, qualitative, non-directive) and the right people (ordinary, normal [young] women). What I failed to recognize was that the problem exists in the structure of the discursive practice of doing research itself, which cannot be simply overcome by good intentions. Another assumption was that feminist practice could somehow exist outside hierarchical relations of power. As Opie (1992) has said, 'textual appropriation of the other is an inevitable consequence of research'.

Empowering research cannot be guaranteed by good principles of procedure or 'soft' research methods. By choosing a 'conversational' research method which did not match these young women's familiar world of interaction with parents, teachers, adults or peers, the research was automatically 'other'. No amount of careful methodological and ethical design and analytic work could make that go away. However, as I have been careful to point out, relations of power are in a constant state of flux. Although power relations are inevitably hierarchical, power itself is not a possession (in this context a possession of the researcher) and neither is it necessarily repressive. In Foucault's formulation it is productive in the sense that in its exercise it produces multiple effects, which produce resistances and create positive spaces.

I have shown how Kate was able to achieve a reversal in the confession discourse by positioning me as the confessing subject. Nadine was able to engineer countless disruptions to interview procedures, which indicated that the research was to be conducted on her terms. Sara positioned herself as a good student/research subject, which enabled her to place definite boundaries around the research relationship, thereby limiting her level of self-disclosure.

I have pointed to the way in which the confession discourse relies on a level of self-disclosure by participants that can result in increased surveillance and interventions designed to 'discipline'. There are also concerns about the commodification of the confession as data, and whose interests this best serves. In the process of doing research the voices and experiences of research participants are mediated first through the recording and transcribing of interviews and later (sometimes much later) in the practice of writing the research. These data are always manipulated and interpreted so that participants sometimes find it hard to recognize themselves in the finished product. While it is the case that all voices and experiences are culturally mediated, this type of research becomes problematic when it is represented as somehow more 'true' or more 'authentic' than other research methods.

However, it should be emphasized that confessing is also a pleasurable practice. We are social beings and we experience pleasure when someone listens to and values what we say. All of the young women welcomed the chance to talk about their experiences: their hopes and aspirations, as well as their concerns, and I welcomed the chance to listen. Speaking out can also challenge some of the commonsense understandings we have about doing empowering research with young women.

Flax (1992) writes about the 'end of innocence' in the postmodern era and some of her comments seem appropriate here;

> ...postmodernist discourses disrupt master narratives of the West and the language games in which terms like freedom, emancipation, or domination take on meaning...no longer serving as the neutral instrument of truth or the articulator of a homogeneous 'humanity's' best hopes, what authorizes the intellectual's speech? ...we can no longer sustain the illusion or the hope that 'true' knowledge is only sought by the virtuous, is a priori generated by the good and when put into practice will only have the beneficial results we intend...All epistemological talk is not useless or meaningless, but a radical shift of terrain is necessary.

It is of course profoundly disconcerting to realize that there is no certain knowledge about how we as researchers should act for the benefit of others; to come to know that our innocence is corrupt. But although everything is dangerous it is not necessarily bad. Flax urges us to 'analyze what has occurred within different discursive practices' and to 'articulate why one set of practices appears to be preferable for certain pragmatic purposes'. Pragmatic action may be the best we can hope for. This is, after all, a much more modest but perhaps ultimately more do-able project than the more ambitious projects we may have previously mapped out for ourselves.

REFERENCES

Alcoff, L. (1988) Cultural feminism versus post-structuralism: the identity crisis in feminist theory. *Signs* 13(3), 405–36.

Alcoff, L. (1991) The problem of speaking for others. *Cultural Critique* Winter, 5–32.

Alcoff, L. and Gray, L. (1993) Survivor discourse: transgression or recuperation? *Signs* 18(2), 260–90.

Davies, B. (1989) *Frogs and Snails and Feminist Tales: Preschool Children and Gender*, Allen and Unwin, Sydney.

Davies, B. (1991) The concept of agency: a feminist poststructuralist analysis. *Social Analysis* 30, December, 42–53.

Ellsworth, E. (1989) Why doesn't this feel empowering? Working through the repressive myths of critical pedagogy. *Harvard Educational Review* 59(3), 297–324.

Flax, J. (1992) The end of innocence, in *Feminists Theorize the Political*, eds J. Butler and J.W. Scott, Routledge, New York and London, pp. 445–63.

Foucault, M. (1977) *Discipline and Punish: the Birth of the Prison*, Pantheon Books, New York.

Foucault, M. (1978) *The History of Sexuality, Vol. 1, An Introduction*, Pantheon Books, New York.

Foucault, M. (1980) Truth and power, in *Power/Knowledge: Selected Interviews and Other Writings 1972–1977*, ed C. Gordon, Pantheon Books, New York, pp. 109–33.

Foucault, M. (1983) The subject and power, afterword to *Michel Foucault: Beyond Structuralism and Hermeneutics*, ed H. Dreyfus and P. Rabinow, University of Chicago Press, Chicago, pp. 208–26.

Gore, J. (1993) *The Struggle for Pedagogies: Critical and Feminist Discourses as Regimes of Truth*, Routledge, New York and London.

Henriques, J., Hollway, W., Urwin, C. *et al.* (1984) *Changing the Subject*, Methuen and Co. Ltd, London.

Hollway, W. (1984) Gender difference and the production of subjectivity, in *Changing the Subject*, eds J. Henriques, W. Hollway, C. Urwin *et al.*, Methuen and Co. Ltd, London, pp. 227–63.

hooks, b. (1989) Feminist politicization: a comment, in *Talking Back: Thinking Feminist, Thinking Black*, ed b. hooks, Boston, South End.

Leahy, T. (1994) Taking up a position: discourses of femininity and adolescence in the context of man/girl relationships. *Gender and Society* 8(1), 48–72.

Lenzo, K. (1994) Reinventing ethos: validity, authority, and the transgressive self. Paper presented at the 78th Annual Meeting of the American Educational Research Association, New Orleans, April 1994, pp. 1–16.

McHoul, A. and Grace, W. (1993) *A Foucault Primer: Discourse, Power, and the Subject*, Melbourne University Press, Carlton, Victoria.

McLaren, P. (1989) *Life in Schools: An Introduction to Critical Pedagogy in the Foundations of Education*, Longman, New York and London.

McNay, L. (1992) *Foucault and Feminism*, Polity Press, Cambridge.

Oakley, A. (1981) Interviewing women: a contradiction in terms, in *Doing Feminist Research*, ed H. Roberts, Routledge, pp. 30–61.

Opie, A. (1992) Qualitative research, appropriation of the 'other' and empowerment. *Feminist Review* 40, Spring, 52–69.

Roman, L. (1987) *Punk Femininity: The Formation of Young Women's Gender Identities and Class Relations Within the Extramural Curriculum of a Contemporary Subculture*. PhD thesis, UMI Dissertation Information Service.

Sawicki, J. (1991) *Disciplining Foucault: Feminism, Power, and the Body*, Routledge, New York and London.

Scott, J. W. (1991) The evidence of experience. *Critical Inquiry* Summer, 775–97.

Sharpe, S. (1994) *Just Like a Girl: How Girls Learn to be Women From the Seventies to the Nineties*, Penguin, Ringwood, Victoria, Australia.

Smith, D. (1988) Femininity as discourse, in *Becoming Feminine: the Politics of Popular Culture*, eds L.G. Roman and L. Christian-Smith, Falmer Press, London, pp. 37–59.

Tait, G. (1993) Reassessing street kids: a critique of subculture theory, in *Youth Subcultures: Theory, History and the Australian Experience*, ed R. White, National Clearinghouse for Youth Studies, Hobart, Tasmania, pp. 1–6.

Taylor, S. (1993) Towards a feminist classroom, in *Texts of Desire*, ed L. Christian-Smith, Falmer Press, London, pp. 126–44.

Walker, J. C. (1988) *Louts and Legends: Male Youth Culture in an Inner-City School*, Allen and Unwin, Sydney.

Weedon, C. (1987) *Feminist Practice and Poststructuralist Theory*, Basil Blackwell, Oxford.

Willis, P. (1977) *Learning to Labour: How Working Class Kids Get Working Class Jobs*, Saxon House, England.

CHAPTER 6

Memory-work: process, practice and pitfalls

Glenda Koutroulis

This chapter on memory-work forms part of a study about menstruation which I undertook as a doctoral candidate. Components of the memory-work process are explained; emphasis is placed upon the practical application of methodological aspects, and the experiential and interactive dynamics of those who participated in the memory-work collective. I use the terms collective and group interchangeably to mean the same thing – a body of people who came together for the common purpose of 'doing' memory-work. Individual collective members are referred to by pseudonyms.

THEORETICAL UNDERPINNINGS OF MEMORY-WORK

Memory-work was first developed by Haug (1987) in a collective study of female sexualization. Designed to bridge the gap between experience and theoretical understanding, the aim of the research by Haug and her colleagues was to understand the social construction of individual identity. In so doing, they set out to:

> ...investigate the organization of bodily activities; the ways in which the body itself and the feelings in and around it have arisen historically; and the ways in which this relates to our insertion into society as a whole. (Haug, 1987)

The theoretical origins of memory-work grew out of a resistance to dominant cultural ideologies which, Haug argued, rendered women largely invisible in the public domain through exclusion and subjugation. Haug begins with the premise that experiences of life contain contradictions, and as social relations stand today, particularly for women. She proposes that during the process of socialization women inscribe themselves into social structures so as to live in a relatively non-contradictory way.

Life's events are restructured or dealt with in a way that minimizes the contradictions, making way for social action but at the same time distorting reality by mechanisms such as self-delusion, the avoidance of conflict, and not confronting issues face to face. Haug believes that life for women becomes a series of compromises in an attempt to find meaning and fulfilment within a given social space.

Haug's discussion portrays women as victims of a repressive social environment. She places a value upon women becoming autonomous rather than remaining heteronomous, and moving from a state of unhappiness toward fulfilment. Haug (1992) argues that oppressive structures can only survive as long as those who live within them reproduce them. In her view, 'being a victim is also an action, not a destiny' and actions contain an element of acquiescence. When Haug talks of socialization she is referring not simply to a process of being moulded/shaped by others, but to a process that requires acquiescence at every stage. Thus, Haug claims women are players in the shaping and reinforcing of those same social structures in which they are imprisoned. She concludes that subordination of the self to social structures, even if not consciously determined, is participating in the cementing of those structures.

Having actively participated in becoming what we are (subjectified), Haug argues we can therefore change what we are. Thus, memory-work becomes a vehicle for bringing about desired change. What becomes of interest to Haug is the potential that memory-work has for liberation. She says memory-work 'must be seen as an intervention into existing practices...[and] our intervention is itself an act of liberation' (Haug, 1987).

MEMORY-WORK: THE STEPS

The subject and object of the research are one and the same person, and memories are the objects as well as the instruments of research. That is, 'the researcher is identical with the object of research'(Haug, 1992). Thus, memory-work:

> ...begins with the particular memories of individual people, memories which they take to be their own personal stories, which belong to them, are of them and which signify who they are. They are central to their sense of self, their subjectivity. (Davies, 1990a)

Haug's approach to the research is that it is a collective endeavour with each member actively participating in the research process. This includes, among other activities, the sharing of ideas, workload, knowledge and analysis. The idea of collective research is a pragmatic initiative in regard to work distribution but, as importantly, it exhibits what Haug calls a move away from the ideology of individualizing and atomizing life's experiences.

There are a series of steps involved in carrying out memory-work, and particular criteria to consider when using the method. The collective meets on a regular basis. One of the first initiatives is to collectively decide on a theme to write a memory about. Haug contends that the theme, chosen collectively, makes it generalizable and significant for the socialization of wider groups. Each person writes a memory of her or himself in the third person. Attention is given to fine details, uncensored, disregarding any thoughts of relevance; recall may be facilitated by focusing on a particular sound, sight or smell. At the next meeting the memories are read to the group, who then analyse and theorize them through a cross-sectional approach. This may be a lengthy process, taking place over several meetings. Analysis focuses on comparing memories, decoding language, silences, contradictions, generalizations and discussing ideas from popular culture; at the same time, efforts are directed toward resisting psychoanalysis, interpretation, value judgements, explanation and biographical accounts. The final step is that each person rewrites her or his memory which, like the initial memory, is collectively analysed and reappraised.

CONSTRUCTION OF THE COLLECTIVE

There are no rules for selecting who to include in a memory-work group. It is likely that the research question will influence who is selected and, in turn, who agrees to participate. There is a variance in opinion about the make-up of a workable group by those who have experience in using the method. Haug (1987) asserts that 'the more diverse the backgrounds and present occupations of members of the collective, the more far-reaching the insights gained into socialization in general'. Crawford *et al.* (1992) are in agreement that a heterogeneous group is more likely to have wider relevance. Kippax (1990), on the other hand, finds that friends are good to work with when undertaking memory-work, which is suggestive of a more homogeneous group than that described by Haug and Crawford *et al.*

Our collective began with eight women, including myself, five of whom were my friends. I was particularly keen to work with friends and in part had chosen memory-work as my method because of this. It meant I could select a group of women that I already had an established relationship with, suggesting a level of comfort and trust with self-revelation that I might not find with a group of strangers. Additionally, involving friends in the research provided an elite avenue for confirming the importance and value I placed on each friend's experiences, views and feelings.

Having said that the collective began with eight members, it finished the project with six members, as following the third and fifth meetings respectively, two women withdrew.

Some may consider 'researching' self and friends unusual, and the question of ethics in doing so needs to be addressed. One ethical dilemma is that friendship invites disclosure (Cotterill, 1992), and as with other close research relationships, great quantities of intimate and extraneous information may be revealed (Cotterill, 1992; Ramos, 1989). Sometimes revelations are regretted and Cotterill questions the morality of setting up interviews which encourage painful disclosures. Acceptance of Cotterill's position makes memory-work amoral, because Haug clearly emphasizes that writing memories, and analytically dissecting them, often provokes what is painful or problematic to the individual.

However, retrieving and working on written memories has unknowable consequences. There is a risk that working on memories may be painful and have a destabilizing effect on the individual. Alternatively, working with a difficult memory through reflection may resolve a worrying event (Crawford *et al.*, 1992) and possibly create a resilience within the individual concerned (Haug, 1987). The central issue is to identify where changes have occurred for the individual, points where there has been successful defence against the imposition of others, or where accommodations have occurred. Then, says Haug, the social construction of women's identity will become clear.

INTRODUCING MEMORY-WORK TO THE GROUP

The first meeting of the collective was called to discuss the topic and the methodology. Readings of the methodology were distributed to each member and the meeting began with both a critique and immediate use of the method. All members of the collective participated in or contributed to setting up the rules, shaping the group and shaping the way the material would be used.

Methodological issues of trust and vulnerability, and their effect upon the data gathered, are apparent when Paula says:

> I think to be able to feel vulnerable is not safe,...we need to have that trust and that happens gradually...It's really important that we perhaps talk about that before we start unfolding...The person may just not be able to cope with it, or want to at the time. So, I think it's [the method] really, really powerful, but it's also quite...a force to be taken care of.

The need to secure the care and attention of the group was seen by Paula as necessary before the group could realize its aims. Kippax (1990) proposes that trust is the main criterion for a memory-work group to work well together. The length of time that each individual takes to establish trust and confidence with the group will vary from woman to woman. This being so, any woman's resistance to focus on her own memory for analysis may indicate that she is not convinced her contributions will be treated in the way she desires.

THE THEME

Process – how is the theme chosen?

Through a collective process, a theme that focuses on one situation is singled out for writing a memory about. In choosing a theme, the experience of Kippax (1990) is that 'starting with the obvious is not always helpful'. The obvious question 'is likely to be firmly rooted in popular prejudice' (Haug, 1987), producing what Kippax calls the obvious response – a memory that is over-rehearsed and glib.

Practice – in our collective?

Menstruation had already been determined by me as the theme for investigation, and therefore was not negotiable with the collective. So, the very first step in putting the method into practice saw a point of departure from the rules. The choice of a sub-theme was raised for discussion. The collective very quickly decided that choosing a predefined sub-theme such as menarche, is exclusionary. Narrowing the scope to a particular focus implies that it is a decisive event in one's menstrual history. This again singularizes experiences, assuming that any predefined landmark is as important in one woman's life as it is in another's, and more important than other experiences. The decision was reached to write about 'significant moments'. The scope is broad and reflective, thereby providing each woman with a degree of freedom to decide her own most memorable experience.

The process of discussing menstruation as a significant topic immediately raised debate, which is evident in the following dialogue. Kate commented:

It [menstruation] is not something I want to bring to the surface and wash the dirty linen in public.

This initial comment pointed to the hidden and 'polluting' nature of menstruation, a subject that was to become a theme in the memories.

Jill asserted that the ordinariness of menstruation made it a not-worth-while topic:

It's awful to think though that something one considers kind of a non-entity...I consider all stories about when you get your period and what happened – I find them all very amusing. You know, who cares...I don't want to come in here and have this heart wrenching thing because – oh, she got it on a Friday and there's some significance in that. To me, who the hell cares...Does it have this incredible effect on people, does it? Is this what defines our roles? Is it that big in everyone's lives?

Such statements did not go unnoticed by some of the collective. The ensuing narrative provides insight into the unspoken yet implied non-conviction of the legitimacy of Jill's convictions. Rosa responded to Jill's utterings with 'This is fascinating stuff', to which Jill replied by asking, 'Is it to you?' Rosa then continued: 'We're talking about method and look what's coming out'. Jill replied with 'I think the methodology stinks...Let's talk about our fathers or something like that'.

Here, a major methodological issue is evident. Jill's perception of what constitutes an important topic to research was ruled out of consideration. The implication of this for the method is that selection of group members should have ensured that they all saw the topic as important.

THE WRITING

Process

The next step in the process is to write a memory. Haug argues that to do so is itself a statement that women's lived experiences are worth writing about. Writing is an important step not only because of the positive value that it places on subjectivity, but because women are writing of themselves, 'putting memory into language', instead of being the subject of the writing of others, whose portrayal of them is often objectionable (Haug, 1987). The interconnection of memory and writing, as Greene (1991) sees it, situates both as liberatory, assuming an importance in revising the past:

All writers are concerned with memory, since all writing is a remembrance of things past;...Memory is especially important to anyone who cares about change, for forgetting dooms us to repetition.

Writing in the way that Haug asks involves a transgression of boundaries, exploring new territories, making public what might have always been private, and treating seriously events that might otherwise have been private and dismissed as unimportant. It is because of its importance or significance that something is remembered, and as Haug (1987) states, 'everything remembered constitutes a relevant trace – precisely because it is remembered – for the formation of identity'.

Haug cautions against the use of auto/biography when writing. She says that writing biographically brings a coherence to the memory and hides resistance. At first glance Haug's warning appears contradictory, for writing memories is intrinsically autobiographical, as dissection of the term 'auto/bio/graphy' (self-life-writing)' (Stanley, 1993) shows. Memories are of the self, written by the self, so that analysis of the self is possible.

This being so, I have interpreted Haug's use of the term autobiography to mean writing about the self in the first person.

Thus, Haug emphasizes that memories should be written in the third person, much as a stranger might observe another's actions and then describe the event. She considers this necessary as a means of detachment. As well as distancing, this style of writing gives each person the opportunity to be attentive to the self, and to the smallest and seemingly irrelevant detail. Crawford *et al.* claim that paying attention to detail highlights just how constrained we are by culturally defined notions of relevance. Writing in the third person also serves to denaturalize any existing value judgements (Haug, 1987) and helps with description while working against interpretation, warranting and justification (Crawford *et al.*, 1992).

Practice

Both writing in the third person and writing as opposed to talking were points of focused debate within our collective. However, we fairly quickly conceded that writing in the third person was necessary for the benefits of detail and detachment. The most contentious debate concerned the act of writing. Despite Haug's detailed argument about the importance of writing, some group members said their preference was to use a tape recorder, suggesting that more spontaneous discussion would emerge. This call was resisted, the reasons framed within Haug's meta representation of writing as a weapon; through writing Haug claims women can create a new consciousness, potentially bringing desired change to their lives.

The process of writing presented itself as particularly problematic to Kate who claimed she was at a disadvantage with writing, stating: 'I can't write, I cannot write. I can talk but I can't write'. Any number of theories may be applied to Kate's lack of confidence in expressing herself on paper. However, one explanation is that women have been silenced by being denied the opportunity to express themselves and their history, and have consequently suffered (Haug, 1987). Kate's reaction highlights the possibility that she may believe that 'there is nothing to write about. The everyday of women's lives is...insignificant, unworthy, banal' (Crawford *et al.*, 1992). Kate was finally convinced about the merits of writing, particularly the positive value that writing places on women's expressivity.

THE ANALYSIS

Process

Haug proposes that written memories are ripe for collective analysis through a critical reading. She believes they merit attention, especially as they provide a contextual space to examine ideological language, a basis of domination and subordination that manifests in everyday practices. Haug suggests that the collective concentrate on decoding the memories, giving attention to the gaps, absences, inconsistencies, contradictions, similarities and differences, which should elucidate the social contradictions underlying a given memory.

In an effort to unmask the many forms in which language practices inhibit and distort knowledge, Haug turns to gaps or silence in language, which she says 'is another way of coming to terms with the unacceptable. In people's memories it appears as an absence or rupture' (Haug, 1992). As pointed out by Crawford *et al.* (1992), absences may also indicate the taken-for-granted of everyday life. Illumination of absences by filling in the gaps and drawing out what is not said, and so exposing ideology, is one of memory-work's most challenging tasks.

Analysis invites doubting the memory imbued with a 'false' smoothness:

> Memory is our means of connecting past and present and constructing a self and versions of experience we can live with. To doubt it is to doubt ourselves, to lose it is to lose ourselves; yet doubt it we must, for it is treacherous. (Greene, 1991)

In working toward making sense of and constructing meaning out of memories, analysis sorts out the disjunctions between past and present in an effort 'to uncover the processes whereby the meanings – both **then** and **now** – are arrived at' (Kippax, 1990). Haug says that a central tenet of analysis is attempting to understand collusion in socialization. To trace this theme, she suggests, will lead to knowledge of the way we adjust ourselves into the social world. To this end, 'the task of memory-work is to uncover and lay bare the earlier understandings in the light of current understandings, thus elucidating the underlying conditions of the processes involved' (Kippax, 1990).

CRITICIZING LANGUAGE

Language has been targeted by feminists as a feature of concern and has become the site of political struggle over meaning. For example, the language analyses of Lakoff (1975) and Spender (1985) shows a language rivalling the oppressiveness of social structures, privileging men and silencing women. Haug declares that language, in all its forms, has legitimated women's marginality. As Dallery (1989) says, 'the hegemony of patriarchy is embedded in language'.

Spender (1985) points to the legacy of research whereby 'questions of the relationship between language and power hover at the periphery of research, unable to become central'. Memory-work represents an important shift, bringing language and research together so that language is integrally connected with the methodology.

Central to memory-work, then, is a critique of language. Analysis of language includes exploring the social meanings attached to words and metaphors, as well as challenging the use of clichés. Haug contends that clichés are symbolic of worn and weary language that have the effect of dulling or obstructing thought, analysis and understanding. They do this through feeding into societal expectations by assuming a consensus, and conforming to rigid views of what are considered appropriate feelings and desires for women to possess.

More extensive attention to clichés has been given by Crawford *et al.* (1992) in their study of memory-work and emotions, where they identified five overlapping classes of cliché. For Crawford *et al*, clichés are:

> ...cultural stereotypes – socially prepared ways of seeing, thinking, feeling. Therefore when we use clichés in the text of our memories, we are not only saying something about ourselves, we are also talking in culturally defined ways and thus saying something about what we have internalized of the social order – we are making standard cultural judgements.

Practice

The following is some of the dialogue that serves to illustrate how we tackled the use of language. Kate's assertion is that for her, menstruation is 'matter-of-fact'. But group members embarked on an argument with Kate in that her memory, with its emotive expression of feelings and her language choices, signifies otherwise. For example, Kate says, 'an idyllic time of togetherness was to be marred by the threat of the curse', and on another occasion, 'a planned weekend was almost ruined by the disaster period'. Shane comments: 'There's quite a lot of feeling in there, and a lot of language that would imply that it's not just matter of fact'.

Kate: The process is,...but the inconvenience of it, it's just a matter of going along with it.

Shane: See,'she trussed herself up', it obviously is bigger in your life than being matter of fact like cleaning your teeth. From your story,...it does have a certain impact on your life. Like to even say, 'but I went out anyway'.

Anastasia: The threat of the curse.

Employing the insights of Crawford *et al.*, it is possible that Kate is articulating a cultural imperative that menstruation and happy holidays are incompatible. If Kate has internalized clichés that define holidays as a time when life will be different and 'good', she has also internalized meanings of menstruation that life will be different and 'not so good' when menstruating.

THE REWRITING

Haug considers rewriting of the memories essential for satisfactory com-pletion of the memory-work process. She maintains that rewriting pro-vides the opportunity to articulate and make credible the motives underlying the behaviour of others who feature in the memory. Haug commented that this proved to be an invaluable step in terms of what the group learned. The experience of others is that rewriting is not always productive (Kippax, 1990).

What is gained from the rewriting process may vary from group to group, or from individual to individual. However, collective analysis and the application of theory provides another point of view on what was an individual experience. Thus, theory has the potential to change individual perceptions. Rewriting, then, offers itself as a step toward concretizing the way in which consciousness has been altered by the group.

Within our collective, the outcome of the rewrites achieved what Haug (1992) sees as desirable – the 'wicked' characters in the initial memory had gained some credibility, becoming not so wicked. Rosemary expresses this in the following way:

> I sort of wanted more to understand my mother and may be to see that she had done her best...Whereas before, somehow I felt that I had missed out because she hadn't joined me in this ritual, in this initiation...Maybe it had left me free; it had given me a freedom that I wouldn't have had if she had been more intrusive.

TAKING REWRITING ONE STEP FURTHER

One of the strengths of rewriting the stories emerged in Rosa's account, when through fantasy she represented the possibility of change, more radical than any of us had anticipated. Rosa's rewriting was a deliberate journey to escape imaginatively the boundaries of her life. Rosa's use of fantasy as a narrative device shows a move toward Haug's (1987) urge that writing be 'destructive of culture' rather than reproducing culture where women are subjugated. Fantasy as a strategy to escape a confining culture is not a new narrative device. Walker (1990) details the attraction of fantasy by contemporary women novelists, whose playful depictions of differences among women mark a break with the unquestioning assump-tions about women's identity and place that are characteristic of many novels.

Rosa describes her use of fantasy as an alternative reality:

> Imaginatively changing the inner world is one of the ways we set about reconstituting the self...I thought about the things that had come out for all of us. And I thought if I wanted to rewrite that situa-

tion in order to address the humiliation and the shame and the powerlessness and the unexpressed anger,...how would I go about that.
So I wrote it as if this is how I would like it to have been now, after
going through the collective...I sort of thought about what was there
for everyone and I tried to act back.

Rosemary remarked that 'to a certain extent, this [fantasy] verges on
female 'Raiders of the Lost Ark' or something, [with] a bit of comedy
thrown in'. Writing using Rosa's formula necessitates vision and an ability
to imagine beyond the limits and the boundaries of the everyday life. Rosa
is aware as she is writing that it is her adult voice directing the scene,
rather than the voice she knew as a youngster; and the adult Rosa has a
variety of discourses available to her that were not available to her as a
child.

Haug draws attention to how uncritically we as women accept 'normality', and Davies (1990b) to how we so easily take on board inscribed cultural notions of being. An example lies in the following response to my
suggestion that we all rewrite our memories using fantasy. Shane said:

I can't imagine what changes I'd make apart from standing up in my
story in the middle of the classroom and announcing that I'd just
started menstruating, and everyone singing and dancing.

Shane's statement demonstrates that she quite spontaneously gave an
imaginative alternative to rewriting her story whereby joy and affirmation
are validated. This imaginative scenario contrasts with her written memories that illustrate both the secret thrill and the sense of isolation typified
by having no-one to share the excitement of menarche with.

Rosa opened up another facet to rewriting the memories. She did this
first through the use of fantasy in transcending what was, and secondly
by letting go of the individual experience and rewriting her story out of a
collective consciousness. Rosa had shown that rewriting offers itself as a
possibility to explore what it means to resist the position proposed in the
initial memory. There is a reconstitution of herself produced through the
rewriting. Also, her rewritten memory demonstrates a shift from individual experience into the collectivity of experience: the focus had moved
from how we were different, to the commonality of women's experience.

FURTHER ANALYSIS

The process of writing up the data necessarily involves further thinking
and analysis of that which has already has been debated and analysed in
the group. Kippax (1990) describes this layer of analysis as when groups
'evaluate their own attempts at theorizing'.

Emphasizing collective as opposed to individual effort requires compromise, so that individual styles can be accommodated when presenting written work. When it is an individual, such as a graduate or postgraduate student, presenting group work to which a further level of theorizing has been applied independently of the group, other sets of problems arise.

In part, problems emerge because, from the inception of the memory-work project, the process is defined as one of collective action, whereby all participants collaborate as co-researchers. Anastasia expressed this in the following way:

> We've gone through a process where we've articulated our membership to this group; we haven't said we've come along as subjects to this research project. We've made it very clear that we've come along as equal researchers.

However, as Haug (1992) acknowledges, 'making everyone a researcher is not so simple'.

Discussion of the legitimacy of the title co-researcher being applied to all collective members occurred on several occasions throughout our meetings, and proved to be a source of contention. Rosemary began to expose the contradiction between her and me, both at the level of intellectual input and at the level of commitment, energy and task allocation. She expressed this as demonstrating a qualitative difference between us, arguing that because of this perceived difference she did not consider herself entitled to be called a co-researcher. Rather, that the group was somewhere in between being pure co-researchers and compromising to the demands of the academic institution. Rosemary's stance is reflected in the following passage:

> When I first came my ideal was that we would be pure co-researchers but as time has gone on I have realized that this is not possible, because it would require great commitment and at the end, even though it would be a collective piece of work, you would get the acknowledgment for that because of the [academic] system.

Discussions surrounding ownership of the data inevitably led to vigorous debate. Questions about ownership are associated with competition and capitalist values, such as to whom does it belong, so that ideas are considered intellectual property. Rosa proposed that a useful distinction to make in the ownership debate is if we say 'what I own is my own labour'. For our purposes, it was an important way of recognizing that each of us had put in units of labour and I had put in the greatest number. What I am arguing for is that certain units of this memory-work project, but not the totality of the work, are collective.

NARRATIVE, INTERPRETING AND FURTHER ANALYSIS

Bell (1988) contends that there has been little attention given to narratives that are generated within the research process. Memory-work, concerned with the analysis of written memories, does not specifically address unwritten memories/narrative/anecdotes produced in the process. So, there is a danger that narratives may be seen as an adjunct to the written memories and thus be cast aside. In the group interactions, written memories provided the 'official' data by which memories are privileged in the analysis, and so typically, as Bell might predict, narratives (at first) were freed from analytical scrutiny. In my research I have treated narratives as an inevitable and necessary byproduct of the memory-work process and, as such, subject to analysis.

Narrative evolving from memory-work has lessons to learn from the writing of oral history and autobiography. Smith (1993) details the implications of style on representing the subject of personal narrative. One of the main problems is when the subject's voice is not distinct but contained in the biographer's voice. Smith, like Laws (1990), treats power as the key ethical element in an exercise requiring representation of subject voices. However viewed, narratives bring a distinct set of ethical concerns, some of which I have addressed in another paper (Koutroulis, 1993).

A COLLECTIVE STRATEGY

Haug (1987) points out that within her own collective the intense questioning of memories and selves provoked interpersonal and personal difficulties and 'tensions in group dynamics...which carried the danger of renewed isolation...The disruptive and destabilizing effect of memory-work demands conscious collective counter-strategies'.

Likewise, our collective experienced similar problems, with testy interpersonal exchanges and challenges. This is probably an inevitable consequence of any collaborative exercise, when a group of people with their own range of experiences get together and discuss an intimate topic in a way they might not have done before. Conflict need not be viewed negatively: Butler and Wintram (1991) suggest that along with cohesion, conflict is necessary for the development of group identity.

The need to reflect on the group (debrief) following our meetings was expressed by most members. Debriefing involved articulating the range of experiences emanating from the group meeting and identifying gaps and difficulties, both methodologically and interpersonally. We resolved to build a debriefing strategy into the method, primarily to provide an avenue for addressing all issues (which we called process issues) other than analysis. We set aside specific amounts of time at the beginning and end of each meeting; this could vary at any given meeting, but had to be collectively agreed to. We considered that this strategy would help us to resist being diverted from the analysis and protect against destabilization. Separating the two aspects to our group meetings posed a challenge. However, there were fairly clear lines of differentiation: the analysis was collective and concerned with the memories, whereas 'processing' focused on any combination of interpersonal or group dynamics, and individual or wider issues. So began a concerted effort to integrate processing and analysis without confining attention to one element of the research process at the expense of another.

THE ACCEPTABILITY OF MEMORY-WORK AS A METHOD

Greene (1991) presents memory as a creative liberty-taking shaper of the past, 'far from being a trustworthy transcriber of 'reality''. Memory may embellish, omit, reorder, revise or resignify, as Greene (1991) suggests it does, but in memory-work the boundaries between reality and fiction are not contested and so there is a blatant disruption of an 'authentic truth'. The imperative of memories is not an essential truth; Kippax (1990) points out that 'whether they accurately represent past events or not is irrelevant. It is the process of construction that is important, what is remembered and in what form'. This suggests that the past is a construct, and as such makes reconstruction of the self possible. Thus memory-work, in the way that Stivers (1993) has observed with other forms of personal narrative, raises epistemological issues about social reality as it challenges what counts as legitimate knowledge, and on the interests on which such assumptions rest.

SUBJECTIVITY

In validating memory-work as a sociological tool, Haug (1987), like a number of other scholars, expressed resistance to the belief that subjectivity of experience could not be used as a source of knowledge. She proposes:

> The very notion that our own past experience may offer some insight into the ways in which individuals construct themselves into existing relations, thereby themselves reproducing a social formation, itself contains an implicit argument for a particular methodology.

Haug creatively converts criticisms of subjectivity, such as that individuals cannot 'make 'objective' judgements about themselves' (Haug, 1992) into the object of research. Her concern focuses on exploring how and why 'people alter, falsify and distort their everyday world...[and so] inscribe themselves into existing structures'.

The relative ease with which experience has been authenticated unproblematically within feminist research has come under question. For example, Gavey (1989) is critical of some feminist analyses for privileging experience, creating an aura of experience as authoritatively 'pure and essential'. The idea of an 'authentic' 'pure' experience unmediated by the social, is dispelled in the collective theorizing that takes place in memory-work. The task of collective analysis is to expose the 'inauthenticity' and 'impurity' of experience, so that the embeddedness of ideology becomes clear.

MEMORY-WORK AS A FEMINIST METHODOLOGY

Feminist methodology's main aim is to seek ways of knowing that avoid subordinating women, and in that sense have a political commitment to the empowerment of women (Ramazanoglu, 1992). Feminist groups do this very well, seeking to raise levels of awareness of social structures that keep women firmly implanted in subordinate positions, challenging and confronting in a desire to bring about change (Butler and Wintram, 1991). Butler and Wintram promote the group environment as offering a space to uncover contradictions in life, question ways of knowing, and reframe ideologies and forms of knowledge. Feminist groups have an ethos of action learning and, where no subject is taboo, empower women to become critically conscious (Butler and Wintram, 1991). However, as Hammersley (1992) points out, oppression and emancipation may be appealing concepts but are problematic as analytical concepts because of the array of sources and types of oppression.

On the surface it appears that memory-work is congruent, at least in theory, with feminist principles and fulfils the feminist research character-istics of a consciousness about choice of method; a liberatory outcome; respect for, and exploration of, women's knowledge and their experience; contextualizing individual women's stories in relation to other women's stories; a shared enterprise whereby the research is structured non-hierar-chically, with all participants being accorded equal status as far as possible; incorporating material not usually discussed in academic disciplines; locating emotions in relation to the research process as a source of insight into the sociological understandings. In addition, memory-work may be termed feminist for its challenge to traditional epistemological construc-tions of knowledge through valuing memory as a rich knowledge source, and for its analysis of gender as a social construction that is amenable to reconstruction.

Despite memory-work being sympathetic to certain feminist research initiatives, my experience leads me to conclude, in the same way as Harding (1987) and Peplau and Conrad (1989), that the process of the research is the determining 'feminist factor', rather than the method itself.

As Peplau and Conrad (1989) state, 'any research method can be used in sexist ways'. My own experience was that when I drifted off track, lapsing into a patriarchal mode of conducting research (authoritative, demanding and subjectifying participants), I was very quickly reminded of my role as equal participant by other collective members. Our collective was a group of women with a feminist value orientation, half of whom were versed in research methods. But what of a group of women who do not possess a feminist value orientation and/or are not versed in the most basic principles of feminist research? It is conceivable that if I had facilitated a different group of women, they would have become my subjects. This leaves open the possibility that there is nothing inherent in memory-work to protect it from the wiles of a sexist researcher.

CONCLUSION

There have been differences in how our collective used memory-work but the basic principles that Haug espoused are present. What emerged as important within our collective was: honouring a contract; negotiation and discussion; and striving for an egalitarian approach, with the dismantling of the power differential, or at least a shift in power.

While memory-work seemed to work well with academic groups of women (Crawford *et al.*; Haug) we had to adapt the method to suit our idiosyncratic collective. Logically, then, the method has a flexibility that potentially caters for the unique characteristics of any given group. The adaptations that we made to memory-work were that the topic for research was not a collective decision: rather, it was chosen by me; rewriting using fantasy to show 'what might be'; the addition of the 'processing' step; a further level of analysis carried out by me, independently of the collective but not without their comment.

Collectivity is a central motif in how both Crawford *et al.* and Haug carry out memory-work, including at the various analytical levels, whereas in our collective, although I have maintained contact with members and discussed several issues with them, I am compelled to further analyse the data independently of the group. As long as I continue to draw the collective into further levels of analysis, the less likely I am able to say 'this thesis is my own work'. The implication is clear.

Therefore, questions essential to a critique of the method – ones that may not be resolved – are, how do I, as a postgraduate student, satisfy the demand of an academic institution that this research is my own work, yet at the same time honour what it means to be a member of a collective? Is this method incompatible with higher degree research? Does the very fact that I submit the research to an academic institution for assessment violate the method?

THE TOOL: AS GOOD AS THE PERSON WHO USES IT

Adaptations to or omission of steps in the method lead to the question: When does memory-work stop being memory-work? At a group level, memory-work may be empowering, cooperative, artistic and enlightening. But what if the participants do not share in the theorizing, writing up, or even reflecting on the data for comment? Not to acknowledge the further contribution of the person who chooses what data to extract from transcripts, who situates the data within a theoretical framework, and presents the work in a readable format, to some extent undervalues or even makes invisible the skills required in this process and may change memory-work to the point where it is not a distinctly unique methodology.

Problems with participatory research have not gone unnoticed and Robottom and Colquhoun (1992) identify the tension between the valuing of participatory research and the notion of 'university expertise'. In regard to feminist research, Richards (1993) addresses the effects of feminist writing on analysis of data, drawing out a contradiction that is relevant to my research when she exposes the demotion or removal of the researcher that occurs with the insistence that women speak for themselves. Richards uses memory-work as an example of the 'élite' researcher removal, identifying issues similar to those that I have espoused in my critique and discussion of my own experiences with the method.

I have described elsewhere (Koutroulis, 1993) that while immersed in the memory-work group I did not have a position as élite researcher, and my research skills were subsumed into the group's general approach. Here is a 'Catch 22' situation, because outside the group, as a PhD candidate, I had to take on the position of élite researcher in applying an additional level of analysis to the group analysis (even when I felt the group had exhausted all reasonable analytical approaches). This circumstance left me feeling as if it were now the group who had been demoted, and in some ways that the group promise of collective work had been betrayed. The ideal of equal researchers had been attempted, but not fully realized. The constraints of being a postgraduate student and fulfilling the expectation that I continue to analyse the data independently of the group, indirectly treats the group account as deficient.

On the positive side, the solidarity arising out of the commitment to the shared task of analysis creates a focused environment to express ideas and opinions, as well as to challenge others. Anastasia sums up the benefit of the memory-work research process when she says:

> I don't feel like data's been taken away from me and manipulated and used for your benefit only. I feel like I've been a participant, and by participating, I've had power over what gets said and what doesn't get said, what gets written and what doesn't get written.

While Anastasia was feeling the rewards of shared power, I was having to consider my own values and give serious thought to a method that challenged my belief that university research training accorded me a position different from that of other members of the group. Participating in memory-work with the group as I did taught me otherwise.

ACKNOWLEDGEMENTS

The contribution of collective members – Susie Bunn, Glenys Curry, Rosalie Hearne, Michelle Kermode, Ruth Malpass, Helen Ridgway and Judi Tarn – to the research and to the development of this paper is gratefully acknowledged. The advice and guidance offered by Evan Willis and Lyn Richards is also acknowleged with thanks.

AUTHOR'S NOTE

An earlier version of this paper was presented to the Annual National Conference of the Australian Sociological Association, Adelaide, December, 1992.

REFERENCES

Bell, S. (1988) Becoming a political woman: the reconstruction and interpretation of experience through stories, in *Gender and Discourse: the Power of Talk*, eds A. Todd and S. Fisher, Ablex Publishing Corporation, Norwood, New Jersey, pp. 97–123.
Butler, S. and Wintram, C. (1991) *Feminist Groupwork*, Sage, London.
Cotterill, P. (1992) Interviewing women: issues of friendship, vulnerability and power. *Women's Studies International Forum* 15 (5/6), 593–606.
Crawford, J., Kippax, S., Onyx, J. *et al.* (1992) *Emotion and Gender: Constructing Meaning from Memory*, Sage, London.
Dallery, A. (1989) The politics of writing (the) body: écriture féminine, in *Gender/Body/Knowledge: Feminist Reconstructions of Being and Knowing*, eds A. Jaggar and S. Bordo, Rutgers University Press, New Brunswick and London, pp. 52–67.
Davies, B. (1990a) Menstruation and women's subjectivity. Paper Presented at The Annual National Conference of the Australian Sociological Association (TASA) Conference, Brisbane, Australia.
Davies, B. (1990b) The problem of desire. *Social Problems* 37(4), 501–16.
Gavey, N. (1989) Feminist poststructuralism and discourse analysis. *Psychology of Women Quarterly* 13, 459–75.
Greene, G. (1991) Feminist fiction and the uses of memory. *Signs: Journal of Women in Culture and Society* 16(2), 290–321.
Hammersley, M. (1992) On feminist methodology. *Sociology* 26(2), 187–206.
Harding, S. (ed) (1987) *Feminism and Methodology*, Indiana University Press, Bloomington and Open University Press, Milton Keynes.

Haug, F. (1987) *Female Sexualization: A Collective Work of Memory*, Verso, London.
Haug, F. (1992) *Beyond Female Masochism: Memory-Work and Politics*, Verso, London.
Kippax, S. (1990) Memory-work, a method, in *The Social Sciences and Health Research*, eds J. Daly and E. Willis. Report of a Workshop on the Contribution of the Social Sciences to Health Research, Ballarat, Victoria.
Koutroulis, G. (1993) Memory-work: a critique, in *Annual Review of Health Social Science*, eds B.Turner, L. Eckermann, D. Colquhoun and P. Crotty, Centre for the Study of the Body and Society, Deakin University, Geelong, Vol.3, pp. 76–96.
Lakoff, R. (1975) *Language and Woman's Place*, Harper and Row, New York.
Laws, S. (1990) *Issues of Blood: The Politics of Menstruation*, Macmillan, London.
Peplau, L. and Conrad, E. (1989) Beyond nonsexist research. *Psychology of Women Quarterly* 13, 379–400.
Ramazanoglu, C. (1992) On feminist methodology: male reason versus female empowerment. *Sociology* 26(2), 207–12.
Ramos, M.C. (1989) Some ethical implications of qualitative research. *Research in Nursing and Health* 12, 57–63.
Richards, L. (1993) Researching families: new challenges to old methods, in *Family Sociology, Developing the Field*, ed L. Arnaulg, Public Institute for Social Research, Oslo.
Robottom, I. and Colquhoun, D. (1992) Participatory research, environmental health education and the politics of method. *Health Education Research* 7(4), 457–69.
Smith, S. (1993) Who's talking/who's talking back? The subject of personal narrative. *Signs: Journal of Women in Culture and Society* 18(2), 392–407.
Spender, D. (1985) *Man Made Language*, Routledge and Kegan Paul, London.
Stanley, L. (1993) The knowing because experiencing subject: narratives, lives, and autobiography. *Women's Studies International Forum* 16(3), 205–15.
Stivers, C. (1993) Reflections on the role of personal narrative in social science. *Signs: Journal of Women in Culture and Society* 18(2), 408–25.
Walker, N. (1990) *Feminist Alternatives: Irony and Fantasy in the Contemporary Novel by Women*, University Press of Mississippi, Jackson and London.

CHAPTER 7

Existing sources and the methodological imagination

Allan Kellehear

What has happened to methodological diversity in health social science research? Where has it gone? Interviewing or surveying methods are now so favoured in health social science research that they are overwhelmingly identified with it. Talking to people is widely seen to be 'real' research. Even the multidimensional strategies of action research and ethnographic methods have commonly privileged this stock-in-trade of the academic researcher – talk. In the context of these values, other methods such as the study of existing sources are frequently viewed as remote, abstract, historical or limited.

These attitudes create a self-fulfilling prophecy amoung health social science workers. On the one hand, they limit the methodological imagination by restricting its view of other methods to narrow and simple stereotypes, thereby reducing their appeal; on the other hand, when the few who do venture into the study of existing sources finally do so, their attempts often reflect their narrow understanding and experience of the possibilities of these methods. Ironically, this limited or abstract use of the method lends support to the stereotypes by providing evidence of its apparent limitations. And so the problem turns full circle.

The aim of this chapter is to encourage a rethink about other methods, particularly the study of existing sources. It is true that this method has often been employed in limited ways, but this is a problem about its current use and not its genuinely rich and diverse ongoing possibilities for health research. If we are to break away from our overreliance on talk-only methods, to develop greater imagination in our research designs, we must take a fresh look at the methodological possibilities available. By providing complementary, comparative and/or contextualizing insights, the study of existing sources is one option which can take us beyond the findings gained through direct methods such as interviews or surveys. In this chapter I will attempt to demonstrate how.

First, I will provide some preliminary support for the view that the study of existing sources has been employed in narrow ways in health research. Then I will demonstrate, through a recent study of the near-death experience (Kellehear, 1996), how the examination of existing sources may be imaginatively employed to further a research area, particularly one dominated by interview data.

HEALTH SOCIAL SCIENCES AND THE STUDY OF EXISTING SOURCES

What, exactly, is the study of existing sources? Existing sources is a phrase that traditionally refers to any written or audiovisual records, such as archive data. A wide range of items may be included here: existing statistical data sets from previous research; registry data; personal diaries; letters; library books and periodicals; company or government records; newspapers; music; photographs and film; census data; or even art work. More recently the phrase has been expanded to include television and material culture. Material items such as motor cars; housing styles; interior decor; physical design of social spaces in shops or schools; household refuse; graffiti; cemeteries; and personal items such as clothing or jewellery are just some of the items included here. There are a number of analytical strategies that one can employ to analyse these data sources, almost all of them forms of content analysis.

When someone else's statistics are analysed this is usually referred to as 'secondary analysis', basically because the data have not been collected by the analyst. In this way also, such work is not viewed as 'empirical'. However, when the actual data sets are collected by the person who also analyses the data, as in content analysis of television, graffitti or household garbage, the research is seen to be empirical.

Away from the well known practice of secondary analysis of other people's statistics, content analysis may be highly structured, hypothesis testing and quantitative. At other times it may be more qualitative, as when themes are inductively collected from examination of recurrent features of social surroundings, objects or the literary texts of diaries or letters. Further than this, however, textual material can be examined semiotically by looking for underlying or hidden themes or ideas which appear to control the appearance or arrangement of the setting or writing. This is a strategy favoured by many in the cultural, media, communication and women's studies research areas. It is also an integral style of poststructural analysis.

As diverse as these data and their analytic possibilities appear, their comparative presence in health social science research is radically modest. Perhaps predictably, health social science research has interpreted the study of existing sources in narrow and positivist ways. Recently, I examined 10 years of the journals *Australian Journal of Public Health* (also known earlier as *Community Health Studies*) and *Social Science and Medicine* (Kellehear, 1993a) for the presence of unobtrusive research methods. My findings were disappointing. Less than 15%, or about one article in seven, employed unobtrusive methods, and the most dominant expression of this was the study of existing sources. However, the most dominant version of this examination of existing sources was the secondary analysis of statistical records. Typical in that regard was the reanalysis of government statistics, such as those from the Australian Bureau of Statistics.

There were countless studies of hospital, community or infant mortality linked to occupational prestige or income. Morbidity studies also predominated. There were meta-analyses of exercise or road accident data or household expenditure. Finally, there were methodological critiques of existing statistical records, particularly those held by governments. Some studies ventured beyond the confines of social epidemiology but these were few, and in the prevailing context of the other studies sometimes appeared idiosyncratic rather than imaginative. Hall's (1986) study of social class and survival on the *S.S. Titanic* or Jago's (1984) study of 20 years of back issues of the *British Dental Journal* are good examples of this.

Overwhelmingly, the use of existing sources has been conservative in choice of data and in the favoured styles of analysing those data. Perhaps part of the reason for this lies in the desire to emulate the positivist models favoured by the clinical sciences. Or perhaps the lack of methodological imagination in this area is not one of supply but of demand. In that way, journals may be discriminating against the more qualitative contributions.

Although positivist methods dominate the two journals examined, there is no evidence of absolute exclusion. The appearance of Koutroulis' (1990) study of sexism in gynaecological texts used in Australian medical schools is an example, however modest, of the presence of semiotic analysis in the public health literature, such as it is. Whatever the politics of publishing for different methodologies this is only one factor among others.

All the above issues notwithstanding, two points are worth making. First, interview and survey studies seem to dominate the health social science literature. Secondly, the few studies of existing sources appear narrow and positivist, lending support to the rather dismal view that perhaps this is all they have to offer. This, however, is plainly untrue.

STUDYING THE NEAR-DEATH EXPERIENCE

As reported in the medical and psychological literature, the near-death experience (NDE) is a subjective experience described by those on the brink of death. The experience is believed to begin when a person's heart or breathing stops during an accident, illness or surgical operation. During efforts to revive them several sensations might be encountered by the dying person. At first there may be a sensation of leaving one's physical body and viewing the resuscitation efforts as if one is an outside observer. Later, an experience of entering a great darkness, sometimes described as a tunnel, is encountered. During this time feelings of great peace seem to dominate. Still further into the experience the person may find themselves encountering a being of light who facilitates a review – educational rather than judgemental – of their life. Some also report that they meet former friends and relatives who have died. At some point in the experience they decide to return, or are drawn back to their bodies and the scene of their illness or resuscitation.

Not all those who undergo resuscitation report these NDEs but almost half do. Of those who do, some only have an out-of-body experience, others perhaps the tunnel sensation and life review. Still a small minority of people might experience most of the remarkable features just described. Although the experience is quite well known in the parapsychological literature, its recognition in clinical medicine is comparatively recent. Raymond Moody's book *Life after Life* (1975) and the widely attended public lectures of the famous psychiatrist Elizabeth Kubler-Ross have ensured continuing popular and professional interest in the NDE.

There have been several major books on the subject from medical and psychological writers (see, for examples Sabom, 1980; Ring, 1980; Grey, 1985; Morse and Perry, 1990; Blackmore, 1993). Articles regularly appear in journals such as the *British Medical Journal, Journal of the American Medical Association, The Lancet, American Journal of Psychiatry, Social Science and Medicine*, or *American Psychologist*. Furthermore, there has been for 10 years now an interdisciplinary international journal devoted to the study of NDEs, the *Journal of Near-Death Studies*.

Apart from the numerous theoretical pieces written about the NDE to explain its cause and meaning, all the major empirical work on the topic has been conducted by survey or interview. The most famous of these researchers, the US pollster George Gallup, has even published his own work examining the NDE (Gallup and Proctor, 1982). Despite all this intense interest in the subject, and despite the many hundreds of people interviewed and surveyed, our basic understanding of the NDE has altered little since it was first descibed by Moody nearly a quarter of a century ago. As one New York journalist asked me in typical direct style: is there anything new to say about the NDE, apart from tunnels, lights, life review and meeting dead people? Indeed, that remains a good question, for study after study seemed to make a virtue of duplication, almost as if yet more people needed to be asked the same questions because the initial answers or responses seemed so fantastic, so provocative. But 25 years of the one research design is surely quite enough, at least to establish a basic phenomenology for the NDE. Basic description seemed to obsess researchers, partly because there seemed to be a belief that those descriptions might lead to detailed clues to physiological processes – or greater details of life beyond death.

Both materialist and New Age writers sit perched over this description, continually pore over it, seem unwilling or unable to go beyond it. But there are other important questions to ask. Is the phenomenology of the NDE confined to the physical experience of dying? What role do social and cultural influences play in the creation of the NDE? What is its social meaning? What role do academic ideas play in constructing an understanding of these matters? Is there a political rather than a simply religious or psychological meaning to NDEs? These are some of the questions for a sociology of the near-death experience and the ones taken up in the work of Kellehear (1996).

STUDYING THE NDE THROUGH EXISTING SOURCES

Experiences Near Death (Kellehear, 1996) contains research which attempts to develop a sociological examination of the NDE in three ways. First, the NDE is reinterpreted in terms of sociological and anthropological theory. Second, the general community reaction to reports of NDE are described and analysed. Social reasons for these reactions are then developed. Finally, academic reactions to the NDE, their professional attitudes and explanations, are examined and explained in terms of a sociology of knowledge and history and philosophy of science approach.

The argument which drives the above organization is that the NDE should be demedicalized: it is part of the broader experience of personal crisis and should be seen in that context. The basic phenomenology of the NDE is not confined to physical deterioration near death: social and psychological features are found in other areas of human experience and must be explained with these areas in mind.

Community and academic reactions are never culturally neutral. In the case of their respective reactions to the NDE, explanations are shaped by the pattern of conflict over perceived inadequacies in science, religion and institutional authority. For the purposes of this chapter, I will only touch upon sections of the book where the study of existing sources has played an important role in the analysis and development of the book's overall argument. Five examples of the use of existing sources will serve to demonstrate the importance of this method in developing the above insights.

Ethnographic cases

As mentioned earlier, most researchers' response to interest in the NDE has been to interview. Most of these interviews have been conducted with Anglo-European respondents in the USA, Britain and Australia. However, there is a small and highly dispersed set of ethnographic cases of NDE. For example, one Australian Aboriginal case is to be found in an anthropological volume published only in Australia (Berndt and Berndt, 1989). A single New Zealand Maori account is to be found in an Anglo-New Zealand work (King, 1985). There are two accounts of native North American NDEs published in the journal *Omega* (Schorer, 1985), and so on. There are also small interview-based studies in Guam and India.

Ironically, no-one had yet assembled these cases together and compared their features. It is well known that western NDEs are not predicted by sex, social class, religious affiliation or attachment, age or ethnicity – at least in the samples taken. And it was always assumed that although there seemed to be some local variation of imagery in non-western NDEs – native Americans tended to see traditional images whereas urban Anglo-Americans tended to see urban images – the differences were not major.

However, a careful comparison of all the cases did indeed reveal important differences. On their own, each separate ethnographic case did not reveal very much. Taken together, however, they could be grouped together as small cells of NDEs from hunter–gatherer societies and NDEs from societies dominated by archaic religions, for example Pacific cultures. These two groups could then be compared with accounts from the west.

The result was important. The experience of life review seems to be confined to societies such as India, China and western societies. Also, the sensation of being drawn through a dark tunnel was not reported from hunter–gatherer and Pacific cultures. Clearly, culture does play a critical role in shaping the NDE. Societies such as India, China or the UK are dominated by what Bellah (1976) describes as 'historical' religions, where conscience and the life lived by an individual are measures of their social and moral worth. When near death, people from these societies experience a review of their lives.

Conversely, in hunter–gatherer and Pacific cultures the individual identity and sense of worth is closely tied to the community or tribe. There is no sharp division between the divine world and the profane which might encourage the individual to bridge such a gap with good works. An integrated sense of the divine-in-the-world complements the tribal sense of integrated personhood.

Also, although a sense of darkness is widely reported in NDEs the world over, only in societies of high technology and agrarian settlement is the term 'tunnel' used to describe that darkness. This suggests that the tunnel sensation is not a physiologically based psychological experience as suggested by some neurophysiologists, but rather a metaphorical description which is culture based.

Castaway accounts

While reading the newspaper casually one Sunday morning, I happened across a story of two people who were shipwrecked and castaway at sea for several weeks. I was struck by the similarity of their experience to clinical cases of NDE. On returning to work that week, I began searching for other cases of castaway experience. I found several cases from survivors who had written up their accounts in their own books.

It quickly became apparent that castaways experience what I have come to term as social NDEs. When the sequence of events are analysed and the experiences examined more closely, it seems that castaways experience a great sense of loss. This can also be described as a sense of separation which, when combined with a great sense of helplessness and an expectation of dying, can lead to unusual social experiences. The first of these is a review of one's life with or without the aid of another person. The interesting feature of this review is that it is commonly taken from the point of view of 'the other' rather than 'the native' or the usual self. The life is examined as one imagines how others would see it. This is an important feature of the life review in clinical NDE cases.

Also interesting is the high reportage of alleged meetings or encounters with supernatural beings, or even deceased relatives. Sometimes this is merely the report of a sensed presence, but at other times visual experiences do occur. When rescue occurs this is often also unanticipated, since frequently the castaways have given up hope and expect death not rescue. The rescue, and the life subsequent to rescue, is characterized by a whole series of psychological and social adjustments. Life is never the same again for these people. They are commonly more tolerant, more philosophical, more interested in life, other people and learning. Once again, these are common after-effects in people who experience NDE.

These collections of castaway cases opened up a fresh way of viewing the NDE. For the first time, we are able to contextualize the personal experiences of the NDE by seeing them as part of the social experience of separation. I then began to look for other cases and found similar experiences amoung trapped coal miners, shamanic initiates and bereaved people. The trauma associated with separation, feelings of helplessness, expectations of dying and foreign environments regularly led those who experience them to other unusual experiences. These are commonly out-of-body sensations, life review, encountering supernatural or deceased beings, visions of other worlds and experiences of darkness. Unusual circumstances lead to unusual experiences, and death is only one, and not necessarily the most spectacular, example of this.

NDE accounts

Of course, one of the most obvious and plentiful sources of existing data were the NDE accounts themselves. One might think that, given the abundance of these accounts, their interpretation would be rather exhaustive, if not exhausted. This, however, is surprisingly untrue.

There is one special feature of the NDE which, although widely priviliged and reported, is rather remarkably underinterpreted, possibly due to a belief that the interpretation is self-evident. I am referring here to the accounts of the afterlife society reported in some extended NDE accounts. Indeed, some whole books are devoted to such accounts where these contain a fair amount of detail about the afterlife. The question I posed of this imagery was: if these are images of the afterlife society – an ideal, idealized if you like, society – what kind of society is this?

There are a number of possibilities. Throughout history there have been numerous ideas of the 'perfect' society. For example, Cockaygne was the dream society of the peasant, where every gastronomic and sexual appetite would be fulfilled and the gentry would be forced to stand waist-high in excrement for 10 years before they could be eligible for the wonders of this society. Clearly, this was an escapist society where the usual social order was reversed.

Other examples were the Romantics' Arcadian society, one where work was a leisurely activity in Eden-like natural surroundings. Millenarian societies were societies where a God, usually Jesus, would preside over the workings, controlling every activity in His wise beneficence. The Moral Commonwealth was a society based on cooperation. Individuals worked and were motivated by the 'common good'. And, of course, we must not forget the Utopian society. These were ideal societies not because they were perfect (a common misunderstanding of the idea) but rather because they depended on fair and efficient social organization, not individual whims or divine rule.

When NDEs are examined with these models in mind, it soon became obvious that NDE imagery was not immune from politics. NDE images of the afterlife were quite obviously Utopian, privileging organization in their workings. This may also be one reason for the popularity of NDEs, particularly in the media.

Fiction

While browsing volumes at a local book fair I came across Margery William's (1922) classic children's story *The Velveteen Rabbit: or How Toys Become Real*. Turning to the back of the story I read the remarkable account of the rabbit's death. The most intriguing part of this account, for me at least, was that most of the main images of the description matched that of western clinical NDEs! I subsequently ran a search for critical reviews and commentaries on this famous children's story. Interestingly again, I found among several key commentaries disappointment and criticism of the rabbit's death scene. In effect, this was a psychoanalytical and therefore materialist response to a non-materialist idea of death, a response identical to one of the key academic responses to clinical reports of NDE.

A key explanation of the psychological features of the NDE is that the ego cannot tolerate the prospect of annihilation and therefore, in the service of this fear, turns on a last minute sideshow of lights, fairy beings and reunions with old friends. This is often described as a defence mechanism and is offered as a culturally neutral 'scientific' explanation based on a taken-for-granted philosophy of empiricism. It also makes two other, rather retrograde, assumptions. First, meanings of death which feature survival of the self must necessarily indicate a denial of death, and second, concepts of death other than materialist ones must be psychologically defensive in origin. A good argument can be mounted to show that both of these assumptions are faulty.

When the story of *The Velveteen Rabbit* is subjected to a simple narrative analysis, as opposed to psychoanalysis, and the death scene is placed in the context from which it arises, the meaning of the scene has little to do with denial. The main theme of the story is that 'real' does not have anything to do with material appearances. In fact, appearances deceive. Worthwhile relationships must transcend physical looks. The depth and strength of love takes time and cannot be hurried. As the Skin Horse advises the Velveteen Rabbit:

> Generally, by the time you are Real, most of your hair has been loved off, and your eyes drop out and you get loose in the joints and very shabby. But these things don't matter at all, because once you are Real you can't be ugly, except to people who don't understand. (Williams, 1922)

The death scene of the rabbit is designed as a literary device, a licence to continue this theme one final and dramatic time. Death does not end love, because love is not wholly dependent on the material. This is a far more complex social idea for children and psychoanalytically minded adults to grasp than the simple contextless idea of denial. But the semiotic analysis of *The Velveteen Rabbit* as fiction permits us to see that the task of reinterpreting meanings of death is important politically in social science, lest one idea is allowed to dominate and control all others. When this dominance goes unchallenged, authoritative ideas become authoritarian and simple academic ideas become menacingly ethnocentric.

Neurophysiological literature

Most people view literature as something to consume. The major issue confronting consumers is the question of whether one agrees with the author(s) or not. In the NDE literature the theories about the NDE as hallucination come from neuroscience. The common academic practice is to read for the details and decide the credibility of the thesis on the basis of the 'evidence'. This approach to the literature is of course quite necessary, if necessarily empiricist in style. I decided to approach the neuroscience literature differently.

I collected together all the principal articles and books which offered neurophysiological theories of the NDE and examined these as one would pieces of fiction. I looked, therefore, at these scientific works as examples of writing. As such I knew that they would employ certain literary devices of persuasion, such as rhetoric and metaphor. But more than this, as most people in the humanities are aware, language itself is no neutral carrier of meaning, and so the language of science in respect to the NDE was also examined.

It is commonly thought, particularly outside academic social science circles, that scientific writing is dry, neutral and esoteric. There is nothing loaded about a chemical analysis and most of the neurophysiological writing was chemical, at least biological. But this is not so. The actual empirical evidence marshalled for a theory of hallucination was rather meagre, much of the writing arguing from metaphor. Theories were often based on other theories. Assertions and arguments were often overinclusive, making generalizations poorly supported or exaggerated. Tracing bibliographies back to their sources produced similar problems, and it became rather obvious that the vehemence of the text exceeded its substance several times over. The only real question was why was the neuroscience voice so shrill and so adamant about the material basis of the NDE when their own evidence was, to say the least, modest?

At this point I was able to look at the decline of medical authority in matters relating to death, particularly over the last 20 years or so. I was also able to re-examine the long-standing conflict that science has had with religion over the centuries, a conflict that re-emerged in the theoretical debates over the significance of the NDE. Finally, I was also able to make some connection to postmodern developments in science and the conservative reaction to challenges here as these were seen to emerge from the discourse over the meaning of the NDE. And all this from a reading of science writing as literary text.

BENEFITS FROM A STUDY OF EXISTING SOURCES

As I believe most readers will readily see, I received three valuable benefits from studying the NDE through existing sources: comparative, contextual and complementary insights.

In comparative terms, my own study was able to supply more than simply a comparison between western and non-western experiences. Other workers had compared, for example, what they believed to be NDEs from highly different societies – China and the USA, or India and the USA, for example. But major differences in social custom do not always indicate major differences in cosmological outlook. It appears that the underlying cosmological attitude, rather than simple differences in religious practice, is the critical influence in shaping NDEs from different cultures.

The comparison between clinical (near death) and social NDEs (expecting to die) led to a successful search and then comparison with social crises (experiences of separation and helplessness). The comparison between community and academic reactions toward the NDE saw lay communities striving for some religious or philosophic context for the phenomenon. Academic communities, on the other hand, sought refuge in a mechanical, materialist concept of consciousness tied to ideas of 'adequate or inadequate functioning'. The difference in approach continues to foster conflict at worst and, at best, to two communities who work hard at ignoring each other's efforts to explain the NDE.

These comparisons provide an important context to our understanding of the NDE, permitting us to move away from a naive empiricism, at first modestly, and then more extensively, toward a social constructionist understanding. This social constructionist perspective is then able to show us how the institutional origins of ideas (science, medicine or religion) are critical in shaping and directing our understanding of things-in-the-world. Meanings do not simply suggest themselves to us in a vacuum: new experiences are seen through the filter of old ones. And so the battle for supremacy of one set of ideas over another is largely a social one.

Both of these insights provide a larger, complementary one. It is often remarked that people were surprised when French sociologist Emile Durkheim (1951) developed an interest in the subject of suicide. Many people then believed, as many do now, that suicide was a private, personal problem, but by providing comparative analysis of the suicide statistics with past times and places, Durkheim was able to show that the private act has a wider context and social significance. Religious meanings and the economic fortunes of nations played important and influential roles in private acts and meanings.

This clever and thoughtful use of existing sources – in this case statistics – allowed a fresh and complementary perspective to shed light on what had previously been regarded as solely the province of psychology. The study of existing sources in the analysis of phenomena near death, I believe, has achieved something quite similar. There is little doubt that the NDE is a private psychological experience, especially from the point of view of those who undergo these remarkable experiences. But a comparative dimension has provided a social and cultural context that has enabled us to see such experiences as part of a wider reservoir of human experience. We are, once again, in a position to complement the insights of medicine and psychology with those of sociology and anthropology, because once again we are able to look beyond and behind the private meanings of individuals.

SOME PARTING SUGGESTIONS

The above insights are not easily obtained by interviews or surveys, espe-cially since the interest areas were so broad-ranging. Although the existing sources in this area were not particularly obvious to me initially (this work and realization took several years to unfold), to have approached these issues with direct methods would have been unnecessarily complex.

Nevertheless, it is one thing to sing the praises of the study of existing sources in retrospect. It is quite another for other researchers to follow what must often seem a highly idiosyncratic path. With this problem in mind, I offer three general suggestions that might be helpful in thinking about the study of existing sources for your own work.

First, I think it is important to get to know your own institutional library, not as a source of reference material but as a source of data. It is important to know what types of archival and record holdings the library has that may complement one's own interests. Valuable to know will be the type and extent of government records/statistics, newspapers, physical artefacts, photograph and film holdings. The 'library tour' is vital to acade-mic staff every bit as much as for the students they send there every year.

It is a good idea also to familiarize yourself with similar facilities in your own city. For example, one of the larger public libraries in my own city has a video disc service for photographs: using a compact disc terminal one can search old photographs by selecting keywords such as 'rural', or 'domestic life' or 'immigrants' and so on.

The second important step in gaining an overview of available existing sources is to examine some guides to these. Among works of interest here are Plummer's (1983) *Documents of Life*; Scott's (1990) *A Matter of Record*; Webb *et al.*'s (1981) *Non-Reactive Measures*; Kellehear's (1993b) *The Unobtrusive Researcher*; Dale *et al.*'s (1988) *Doing Secondary Analysis*; and Stewart's (1984) *Secondary Research*. Obviously other general guides, which are often methodological guides as well, can be found by searching key-words in the library catalogue, such as 'unobtrusive research', 'secondary analysis', 'content analysis', 'non-reactive measures', or 'archival' or 'docu-ment' research.

Even more specific as a guide to sources are directories of information. A chat with any librarian can lead you to these, but for an example see Codlin's (1990) *Directory of Information Sources in the UK*. Codlin lists over 5000 organizations which make information and records available to inter-ested people. Incidentally, there are also similar guides to existing statisti-cal data sets, from both government and private research sources.

Finally, of course, there is your own methodological imagination. Valuable sources may not always be obvious, as one can see from my dis-covery of castaway accounts or the children's story *The Velveteen Rabbit*. To some extent, a bit of lateral thinking can help create one's own serendipity. It is important to compare the literature of your interests with seemingly unrelated literature. Compare, for example, the social science literature of travel and tourism with that of AIDS symbolism in medical journals.

C. Wright Mills (1959), in *The Sociological Imagination*, recommended that one should keep files of one's own writing, notes or articles on different interests, and from time to time mix some together randomly to stimulate theoretical imagination. This apparently strange process can be quite fruitful in the search for new connections and ideas. And, given the present state of methodological preferences in health studies, a few new connections and ideas might be warmly welcomed and encouraged.

REFERENCES

Bellah, R.N. (1976) *Beyond Belief: Essays on Religion in a PostTraditional World*, Harper and Row, New York.

Berndt, R.M. and Berndt, C.H. (1989) *The Speaking Land: Myth and Story in Aboriginal Australia*, Penguin, Ringwood.

Blackmore, S. (1993) *Dying to Live: Science and the Near-Death Experience*, Grafton, London.

Codlin, E. (ed) (1990) *Directory of Information Sources in the UK*, Aslib, London.

Dale, A., Arber, S. and Proctor, M. (1988) *Doing Secondary Analysis*, Allen and Unwin, London.

Durkheim, E. (1951) *Suicide: a Study in Sociology*, The Free Press, New York.

Gallup, G. and Proctor, W. (1982) *Adventures in Immortality*, Souvenir, London.

Grey, M. (1985) *Return from Death*, Arkana, London.

Hall, W. (1986) Social class and survival on the S.S. Titanic. *Social Science and Medicine* **22**, 687–90.

Jago, J. (1984) To protect the public: professionalism vs competence in dentistry. *Social Science and Medicine* **19**, 117–22.

Kellehear, A. (1993a) Unobtrusive research in the health social sciences. *Annual Review of Health Social Sciences* **3**, 46–59.

Kellehear, A. (1993b) *The Unobtrusive Researcher: a Guide to Methods*, Allen and Unwin, Sydney.

Kellehear, A. (1996) *Experiences Near Death: Beyond Medicine and Religion*, Oxford University Press, New York.

King, M. (1985) *Being Pakeha: An Encounter with New Zealand and the Maori Rennaissance*, Hodder and Stoughton, Auckland.

Koutroulis, G. (1990) The orifice revisited: women in gynaecological texts. *Community Health Studies* **14**, 73–84.

Mills, C. W. (1959) *The Sociological Imagination*, Oxford University Press, New York.

Moody, R. A. (1975) *Life after Life*, Mockingbird, Covington.

Morse, M. and Perry, P. (1990) *Closer to the Light*, Souvenir, London.

Plummer, K. (1983) *Documents of Life*, George, Allen and Unwin, London.

Ring, K. (1980) *Life at Death: a Scientific Investigation of the Near-Death Experience*, Coward, McCann and Geoghegan, New York.

Sabom, M. B. (1980) *Recollections of Death: a Medical Investigation*, Harper and Row, New York.

Schorer, C. E. (1985) Two native North American near-death experiences. *Omega* **16**, 111–13.

Scott, J. (1990) *A Matter of Record*, Polity Press, Cambridge.

Stewart, D. (1984) *Secondary Research: Information, Sources and Methods*, Sage, Beverly Hills.

Webb, E., Campbell, D., Schwartz, R. *et al.* (1981) *Non-Reactive Measures in the Social Sciences*, Houghton Mifflin, Boston.

Williams, M. (1922) *The Velveteen Rabbit: or How Toys Become Real*, Doubleday and Co., New York.

CHAPTER 8

Opening up awareness: researching nurses' attitudes towards dying patients

David Field

INTRODUCTION

Qualitative methods of research have been accepted and used by nurses for some time and are increasingly being viewed as a useful component within health services research. Unstructured interviews are one of the methods of qualitative research which are frequently used, although not always with a full understanding of the principles of qualitative research. Without such an understanding the appropriate use of this method is unlikely. In this chapter I attempt to demonstrate both the importance of applying the basic principles of qualitative research when using unstructured interviews and the usefulness of this method by drawing upon my research into nurses' experiences of nursing terminally ill patients (Knight & Field 1981; Field 1984, 1989a, b).

My research developed out of my involvement in teaching about death and dying. This was a topic which evidently aroused both great interest and some anxiety among medical and nursing students, but the bulk of the material available referred to US experiences and there was little empirical evidence about how death and dying were handled in the UK. One motivation for the research was to see whether it was possible to generalize from the American experiences to those in the UK. The hope was that the research would inform further teaching in this area. A second factor was that much of the work in the area derived from psychological and psychoanalytic perspectives. However, three sociological studies in the USA (Glaser & Strauss, 1965a, b, 1968; Quint, 1968; Sudnow, 1967) demonstrated the central importance of the social organization of hospital work to the care of those who were dying, in particular the ways in which communication of information about prognosis was handled by staff were identified as being central to the experiences of dying patients, their relatives and hospital staff. This finding had been confirmed by a British study (McIntosh, 1977). As a sociologist I wanted to discover whether, as more recent US research suggested (Greenwald & Nevitt, 1982), patterns of communication about terminal illness were in fact more 'open' and whether the social organization of nursing work in different settings influenced such communication. The aim here was to demonstrate the importance of social organization in facilitating or hindering nursing work.

CHOICE OF METHOD

One of the main strengths of the unstructured interview method is that it is good for developing descriptive and in-depth 'case history' type material, and for 'allowing the subject to speak for themselves'. An example of such material is the following extract from an interview with a staff nurse, where she describes her contrasting experiences of nursing dying people on her current and previous wards:

We had a patient who was here over a year – and we were all very close to 'C'. I saw him from when he came in, to getting really better, then going down again. It was awful because there was nothing I could do – I just had to sit and hold his hand. At that time we were all taking it in turns to sit with him as long as we could 'cos we just didn't want him to die on his own. Nobody wanted just to go in and find him dead. Which I think goes for most of the patients that you know are on their last legs. You don't want to leave them on their own ... I remember very clearly a patient on geriatrics. I had nursed him on nights, and I went back on to days – he was a double-sided CVA. He was very incoherent. By some miracle he could just whisper words. And at night he couldn't sleep because he was so uncomfortable so I used to spend a lot of my nights sitting and talking to him and holding his hand. When I went back on to days I went behind the curtains – and he was really on his last legs. So I just sat with him and held his hand. And I remember the staff nurse coming in and asking me if I had nothing better to do. So I said 'No. Not at this moment, no'. So she said 'would you mind going and finding something to do?' I remember it so clearly. I really hated her; because this man was dying, I'd been with him all this time, and why should he die alone? All she was content with was giving him BPOs and he still had an enema the day he did die. Well he died that afternoon. I felt awful – this poor little man – and just as I went behind the curtains he just said – he grabbed hold of my arms (he got very little movement in that hand), and he just put his hand on mine and whispered 'I love you'. And then he died in the afternoon. I thought 'well it's all worthwhile' because at least he realized that somebody cared. (Field, 1984, 1989a)

This extract brings to life and vividly highlights some of the important variables which are relevant to the nursing care of dying people in our hospitals. That is, the importance of the senior nurses in defining appropriate work the sentimental order of the ward; the organization of nursing work and the emotional involvement of the nurse with the person who is dying. It also demonstrates the importance of the social organization of nursing work for the care which it is possible to deliver.

Nurses in three settings were interviewed: in a general medical ward (Field 1984, 1989a), in a coronary care unit (Field 1989a, b) and district nurses (Field 1989a). My preferred choice of method was participant observation because I felt that this would provide the richest and most detailed insight into how nurses actually cared for dying patients, and this method was used by a sociology student with nursing experience who worked as a nursing auxiliary on an acute hospital ward (Knight & Field, 1981; Field, 1989a). However, it was not a feasible option for me because I could not commit the long periods of time required due to other work commitments. Unstructured interviewing was therefore chosen as the best alternative because its non-directive and open format would allow me to respond flexibly to what the nurses were telling me and to engage in hypothesis testing and the development of 'grounded theory' (Glaser & Strauss, 1967). As Schwartz and Jacobs (1979) put it, 'qualitative methods, which use natural language, are best at gaining access to the life-world of other individuals in a short time'. Also, the unstructured interview is a good medium for finding out about sensitive, embarrassing or stigmatized subjects, such as caring for people who are dying and emotions about death and dying, by allowing the interviewer to probe in a gentle and non-directive manner.

BASIC PRINCIPLES OF UNSTRUCTURED INTERVIEWING

Unstructured interviews are often used in conjunction with ethnographic methods such as participant observation, and are seen to be based on similar principles. Three basic principles can be identified: the first is that the researcher 'suspends belief' in the normal and taken-for-granted assumptions about the social world and its organization, and instead attempts to discover how people order their behaviour and interpret their world (Hammersley & Atkinson, 1983). Such a setting aside of one's day-to-day knowledge of the world is easier in an alien society, where there are quite evident differences in language, belief and activities, than in one's own soci-

ety. As a sociologist entering the world of hospital nursing it was not too difficult to set aside my beliefs in how the world worked – at least in the hospital setting. A second basic principle shared by both participant observation
and the unstructured interview: as the researcher cannot presume to know
how their respondents make sense of their world, they should avoid applying their own preconceptions and beliefs in interpreting what is being said.
It is therefore important for the researcher to be continually monitoring
themselves in a self-reflexive way in order to ensure that they are not
unthinkingly drawing upon their own perspectives and presumptions.

In both methods the researcher attempts to be non-directive and responsive to new and unexpected information, although the latter inevitably has
a narrower focus of concern and cannot draw on the direct experience of
the researcher as participant in the group's activities. Thus on the coronary
care unit observation was added to the interviewing, although this was not
possible on the general medical ward and knowledge of community nursing work was gained by spending two full days going round with district
nurses, one of whom was attending a terminally ill patient. Active listening
was important: although the interviewer may appear passive, in fact they
must be constantly assessing and monitoring what is being said in order
unobtrusively to steer the interview to areas of interest, to elicit further concrete details, or to follow up new and unexpected lines of enquiry.

A third basic principle, again shared with participant observation, is to
remain faithful to the respondents' accounts. My aim was to gather
detailed descriptive material of the ways in which nurses made sense of
nursing dying patients, without imposing my own concepts or categories
upon such descriptions. I therefore taped the interviews in order to protect against the selective interpretation of what the nurses actually said
(Hammersley & Atkinson, 1983). Discussions with colleagues who had
used this method of data recording extensively and reports of published
research based on taped interviews (e.g. Quint, 1967; Rubin, 1976), indicated no serious difficulties. Certainly it would not have been possible to
record the nurses' accounts fully without the tape recorder, and in any
case I felt that taping would be less intrusive than frantically scribbling
down as much detail as possible. Many of the nurses seemed to forget that
the tape recorder was there, or were unaffected by it, although some did
say that they were aware of it throughout, and on several occasions further elaboration of a nurse's views were forthcoming after the tape had
been switched off. I have subsequently used tape-recorded unstructured
interviews in other academic and policy-oriented research.

PROBLEMS IN CONDUCTING UNSTRUCTURED INTERVIEWS

A number of general problems were encountered which are common to
any interview study. It should be stressed that the success of interviewing

lies not simply in avoiding problems but also in recognizing and coping with those that arise during the course of interviewing. Cicourel (1964) perhaps overstates the case with his remark that '...interviewing is complex and difficult because it necessitates presenting, establishing, and maintaining appropriate and possibly conflicting roles'. Nevertheless, his list of 'unavoidable problems...basic to the interview and routine exchanges in everyday life' aptly identifies these problems and so his analysis is used to provide the framework for the following discussion. For convenience we can divide the problems into those concerned with conducting the interview and those concerned with understanding and interpreting the nurses' accounts.

There were three main problem areas with regard to the interview process itself: establishing and maintaining trust and rapport; unobtrusively controlling the interview; and coping with differing perceptions and meanings.

The success of interviewing is heavily dependent on trust and rapport between interviewer and respondent, and with unstructured interviewing in particular it is necessary to establish and maintain this trust and to maintain the respondent's continuing cooperation and willingness to volunteer information, views and opinions. Good rapport is essential if the respondent is to speak freely and with minimal prompting, particularly where, as in interviews about dying patients, the topic being studied is of a sensitive or delicate nature. Generally it seemed that trust was not a problem in my research: nurses talked openly about 'bad behaviour', criticized other staff at all levels and talked about and displayed their emotions openly. They were clearly not always giving 'safe' and 'acceptable' views. However, maintaining rapport posed some difficulties with regard to maintaining direction and control of the interview, and it was sometimes difficult to maintain the fine balance between remaining non-directive and flexible while retaining overall direction and focus. Digressions and 'irrelevancies' may be the price one has to pay, although sometimes such digressions or 'irrelevancies' in fact pointed me to things I had not realized were relevant.

Control of the interview is vital, but must remain unobtrusive and depends on good interpersonal skills. In the case of my research interviews were generally relaxed and friendly even though, given the topic, they were sometimes characterized by a high level of emotional affect as well. The move from one topic of interest to the next was generally smooth and part of the natural flow of conversation. As all hospital-based interviews and most interviews with community nurses occurred during work time there was an interviewer-perceived time constraint. To a certain extent this restricted the scope of the interviews, although this may well have been a useful focusing constraint. The main consequence was to limit the amount of cross-checking and validating of responses within (but not between) interviews. In any case, as Cicourel (1964) writes, 'checking out responses for consistency and depth may lead to uneasiness and avoidance patterns on the part of the respondent...', and hence threaten rapport and trust.

Another factor relating to control is the status of interviewer and interviewee. In our society these roles are well known (e.g. through knowledge of media interviews) even by people who have not been interviewed before, and there may be both an assumption and acceptance of the idea that the interviewer should be at least directing, if not rigidly controlling the interaction. This may facilitate the interview process by establishing expectations that the respondent, having agreed to the interview, will talk and answer questions. However, other status attributes may intrude problematically: some nurses, especially trainee and enrolled nurses, seemed to regard me as being of a superior social status, possibly because I was a lecturer at the university, and this may have had an inhibiting effect on their responses. The lack of experience of trainee nurses or/and the social class background of some enrolled nurses also seemed to inhibit their responses because they saw themselves as not especially competent. One enrolled nurse, after clearly describing to me how he had gently led a patient and his wife to an understanding that the patient was likely to die from his condition, immediately claimed that he was very poor at explaining things to patients! Whatever the reasons, sometimes the interview process did not proceed smoothly. In such circumstances interviewers need to be very expert in encouraging and allowing people to talk without guiding their responses. This can be very difficult.

An important of feature of unstructured interviewing is the awareness of the researcher of the active part which they and their respondents play in the research process. This aspect is often referred to as 'reflexivity', and self-reflexivity must be consciously used as part of the research process (Hammersley & Atkinson, 1983). The way in which I performed the role of interviewer clearly affected what the nurses told me and so had a bearing on the quality of the material collected. For example, remembering the agenda (a vital aspect of controlling the interview in an unobtrusive way) was sometimes difficult, particularly when I became too absorbed in what the nurses were telling me. To combat this I used a small file card which I could glance at unobtrusively to remind me of the topics I wanted to find out about. While this is useful, there is really no substitute for memorizing one's agenda and actively monitoring it during the progress of the interview. My mental alertness and 'emotional tone' varied with each interview, and this must certainly have interacted with the structural problems of interviewer performance: 'the interviewer cannot possibly check his own responses in detail and follow the testing of an hypothesis during an interview; he is forced to make snap judgements, extend inferences, reveal his views, overlook material, and the like...the interviewer cannot escape from the difficulties of everyday life interpretations and actions' (Cicourel, 1964).

Given the nature of the unstructured interview it is difficult in certain situations to retain a balance between being involved and maintaining detachment. This balance may be particularly hard to maintain when the interviewer identifies closely with the topic being researched and/or with the respondent. For example, it may be difficult for nurses conducting unstructured interviews with other nurses to maintain such balance. A number of researchers, such as Oakley (1981) and Becker (1967), argue that it is not possible to retain detachment, and that in any case to do so is both unethical and detracts from the researcher's ability to grasp the life-worlds of respondents. It is my view that overinvolvement can be personally damaging, can be unhelpful to respondents, may seem inauthentic and/or inappropriate to them, and hinders rather than aids the analytical process. I therefore attempt to remain detached, although not always successfully.

A third general problem was that sometimes the nurses and I had different perceptions and interpretations about what was going on. This was not a major problem as I had chosen the open-ended unstructured interview format precisely to allow for the expression of a range of perceptions and interpretations. As Garfinkel (1967) has observed and documented, people 'read in' and presume meaning and intent within task-oriented (and other) interactions such as the interview, and their responses reveal the meaning they intuit. On a number of occasions nurses would interpret a question, a comment, or even a gesture, in a way not originally intended and many of these misinterpretations proved to be useful in opening up new areas which had not been previously considered, or in amplifying existing categories. For example, it had been assumed that dying patients were different from other types of patients and so initially questions were couched in terms of that assumption. A nurse's 'misinterpretation' revealed that this was not necessarily a valid assumption to make, and led to the exploration of ways in which terminally ill patients were similar to and different from other types of patients. 'Misinterpretation' and 'naiveté' on the part of the interviewer can be used as a way of getting respondents to amplify, clarify or expand on a topic in a non-directive manner, or to cross-check information and on occasion I deliberately used these tactics. I also did so unintentionally.

Nevertheless, unexplicated meanings could be a problem. As Cicourel (1964) notes: 'Both the respondent and the interviewer will invariably hold meanings in reserve; much remains unstated even though the interviewer may pursue a point explicitly'. For example:

DF: What's the problem (causing friction on the unit) now?

CV: What happens is each year you get this cycle. We have a quiet patch and people start niggling, and then they want a unit meeting...when I originally started I was all for democracy and I thought unit meetings would be marvellous, and at the time they were necessary. Now I think they are a waste of time. Despite all the backchat and complaining going on people won't say anything at the meetings. People don't want democracy as long as they're vaguely told or given a choice between a and b(...).

Despite my best efforts it proved to be impossible to discover what the precise point of contention was, although it did become clear that despite the sense of being part of a cohesive team which worked together and supported each other, there were was some disagreement about the running of the unit.

It was not only the nurses who reserved meanings: I also concealed my views on topics of direct research interest (e.g. the nursing process) or which I thought might prove to be contentious (e.g. the value of hospices). This type of interviewer practice has come in for criticism from feminist researchers such as Oakley (1981), who believe that interviewers should reveal their views when asked by respondents to do so. However, there seems to be no sound ethical reason why one should not act in this manner, and such behaviour did not seem to offend the nurses interviewed in the studies under review. On the one occasion when a nurse sought practical advice during the research interview (about communicating about a terminal prognosis with her patient) she appeared happy to complete the interview before engaging in what turned out to be a rather lengthy discussion about her problems with this patient.

MAKING SENSE OF THE DATA

A daunting part of research based upon unstructured interviewing is the analysis of the interview material. How is one to arrive at and justify theoretical explanations and interpretations of the material? How does one select illustrative examples from the corpus of interview material? Analysis is typically laborious and complex, and requires patience, concentration and a good recording system. When interviews are recorded the process of transcribing the tapes is very time-consuming. Estimates vary, but for every spoken hour something in the order of 4–6 hours of transcription is required. Good-quality recording equipment and a proper transcriber (i.e. with variable speed and a foot pedal) make the task more manageable. Given the time it takes, the researcher may be tempted to abandon the full verbatim transcription of interviews. However, full transcription is something which can be useful to the comprehension of emerging patterns. Transcription and data analysis may be especially difficult to keep up with if feedback from the analysis into an ongoing interview programme is planned or required. It is therefore important not to plan too heavy an interviewing schedule. I found more than two interviews a day difficult to manage.

During the interviewing period there are three interrelated activities: interviewing, reviewing completed interviews (and possibly transcribing them), and keeping a research diary or account. I found the second and third elements to be vital for they are central elements in the continual reviewing and checking of the progress of the research. It was in these activities that my research hypotheses emerged and became refined, and new areas or topics for attention became apparent. My research diary contained a variety of elements covering all features of the research programme: factual information about who was interviewed; where and when they were interviewed, together with a synopsis of the interview and any problems or striking features; comments on my moods and self-evaluation of my performance; identification and elaboration of theoretical and descriptive points of interest; self-reflexive comments on my performance; thoughts and speculations. Glaser and Strauss (1967) suggest that the aims of keeping a diary are to encourage self-reflexivity and the exercise of one's analytical imagination, and that it provides a main source for the development of 'theoretical memos' where the researcher tries to flesh out and sharpen up emerging ideas. An excellent example of such work is to be found in the appendix to C. W. Mills *The Sociological Imagination* (1970).

My initial interviews focused on the relation between nurses' experiences of dying patients and patient age, the duration of dying, whether the death was expected and who knew the patient was dying. I was particularly interested in communication between nurses and dying patients and their relatives, and rapidly became interested in the emotional involvement of nurses with such patients. In the process of reading and categorizing the transcript material, and in comparing items within the same category, new interview agenda topics and categories were generated. As these processes continued certain regularities within categories became evident and a category might be judged to be 'theoretically saturated' (Glaser & Strauss, 1967), i.e. no new information was being found. When this happened only a count of the category instance was recorded. Some categories were dropped from the interview agenda and others were modified to elicit more precise and useful information as a result of the ongoing monitoring and review of categories. Extracts from interviews which seemed to be good exemplars of points or problems, or which provided a particularly good description, were also identified at this stage.

In the period between the interviews on the general medical ward and those on the coronary care unit three topics emerged from the more detailed and systematic analysis of the interview material which I decided were worth further exploration, and these were incorporated into the interviews with coronary care and community nurses. One topic, which turned out to be theoretically the most significant, concerned the relationship between the nursing process and care of dying patients: it seemed that the direct and inescapable contact with patients generated involvement and satisfaction for nurses. A second topic was whether nurses thought that patients who were dying were markedly different from those who were not. This topic served to sharpen up the differences between the three settings studied. The third topic concerned the problems and strategies surrounding the achievement of an 'open awareness' about the patient's terminal condition. This was the most important practical issue to emerge, and one which has informed my teaching about terminal care and which continues to be of research interest. To make room for these topics a number of items had to be omitted from the interview agendas for these groups, although this did not prevent nurses from spontaneously introducing them.

When the time came to write up the research material the file cards were reviewed again to identify possible extracts which could be used to illustrate points. Developments in computer technology now mean that this type of analytical work can be done using wordprocessor search facilities or one of the numerous qualitative analysis data packages (Tesch, 1990), which allow the identification and further analysis of keywords or concepts more systematically than by hand. It must be stressed that the researcher still has to identify and tag the concepts and themes – the computer packages only facilitate analytical work, they are not a substitute for it! In selecting examples I took care to quote from as many nurses as possible, and not to quote extensively from only a few. This was one way in which I attempted to ensure representativeness and the validity of my interpretations. The richness of the material generated and the adequacy of its interpretation can only be judged by reference to the published work (Field, 1984, 1989a,b).

There were a number of potential problems in analysing and interpreting the interviews. First, relying upon the nurses' verbal accounts of their work posed the problem of establishing the link between verbally expressed attitudes and non-linguistic behaviour. How valid is taking what people say as a reflection of what they do? The validity or truthfulness of the accounts and descriptions generated by unstructured interviews is sometimes difficult to assess. Respondents may be untruthful either intentionally (e.g. they wish to conceal embarrassing or politically dangerous information) or unintentionally (they mis-recall or forget). There are a variety of ways of checking respondent veracity. One way to protect against some forms of unintentional misrepresentation is to ask the respondents to review their own transcripts, which is what I did, but this is not infallible. The plausibility of the respondents' accounts was important to consider, as was their face validity – did they relate to the questions in an appropriate manner? Was what they said consistent with what is generally known? I also tried to check with other sources of information, e.g. observation, written records and interviews with other respondents. Both within the interview situation and at the data analysis stage it was possible to check for inconsistencies and discrepancies in what the nurses said. However, in the last resort there are no guarantees of validity and the researcher should be as clear as possible about how they went about collecting, interpreting and selecting their research material for final presentation. By making these aspects of the research open to view (Field, 1989b) others may more adequately assess the quality of the research.

Second, the sample sizes are not very large and thus the representativeness and generalizability of the study findings were problematic. However, this was partially overcome by comparative analysis of the responses in the different settings. Indeed, the ability to compare the experiences and attitudes of nurses in the different settings was seen as one of the strengths of the research. The conventional concept of reliability, i.e. the extent to which a different researcher (or the same researcher on another occasion) would elicit the same information, does not make sense to qualitative researchers. This formulation denies the central role of the reflexive interaction between interviewer and respondent in the production of meaning. Rather than eliciting precisely the same data from all respondents, the unstructured interview aims to explore differences and shades of opinion between respondents, to see how far they respond in similar ways, produce similar justifications for their behaviour, and so on. In short, differences between respondents are seen as just as important, and sometimes more important, than similarities between them.

A final difficulty in interpreting my interview material arose from the fact that both transient situationally specific features as well as more durable 'universal' aspects are elicited in interviews. It is important to distinguish these elements from each other, but unfortunately the transient elements are not usually as transparent as in the instance where an interview was interrupted by a cardiac arrest! This example also highlights a second situationally related problem: the choice of interview site is important, but was not always under my control. Interviews conducted in the hospital were subject to interruption, with negative consequences for continuity and mood, and one interview was in fact terminated (after 25 minutes) because two interruptions made it too difficult to continue. Situational variables thus feed back into the control of the interview.

Another problem relating to the situated nature of the interview (which I have mentioned previously) is that commonly shared meanings and background conditions may be so well known, obvious and taken for granted by the participants that they are not conveyed to the interviewer. This may be less of a problem with structured interviews – although it is always a problem in any interview – but it is central to the unstructured interview. I never became fully conversant with all of the technical jargon used by nurses. More importantly, although I was concerned with and enquired about the structure and organization of nursing work, I could not assess all the changes in working conditions which affected the nurses. For example, on a follow-up visit to the coronary care unit to discuss the first draft of that research paper I discovered some new information. I had become aware of the concern of nurses about the high level and steady increase in the number of 'unsuitable' admissions to the unit during the study period. However, I had not fully related these concerns to the more general underlying structural problem of control. It was not simply a matter of restricting such admissions, but also concerned the inability of the nurses to exercise their expertise with such patients.

These problems are fairly typical and show the importance of combining the unstructured interview with other methods of data collection, such as observation and the review of written records whenever possible. Denzin (1989), among others, suggests that 'triangulation' of data using a number of different methods is highly desirable.

ETHICS AND RESPONSIBILITIES

I want to end by talking about the responsibilities one has to oneself and to those one studies. There is not much point in doing research if the results do not reach the appropriate groups. Indeed, one of the responsibilities of any researcher is to ensure that his or her research is used – how otherwise can the intrusion into respondents' lives be justified? One way to publicize research activity is to present papers and posters at conferences and to publish in the journals. As the academic audience was not the only, nor even the main, audience for the results I targeted nursing journals and presented my work to national and local nursing conferences. I also sent copies of my analysis to the general medical ward and the coronary care unit, although as the community nurses did not work in one unit I could not do this with them. I also used my findings in my teaching to medical students and nurses. Finally, I managed to secure a contract for a book which pulled together all the research into one easily accessible (and cheaply priced) form.

A second important responsibility to respondents is to do them no harm, neither during the research process nor as a result of making the results of research known. In this context the use of covert participation on the acute surgical ward came in for severe criticism (Johnson, 1992). Our justification for adopting this approach was that to openly act as a participant observer would have compromised the research by changing nursing behaviours. Our main interest was patient care, and this could best be observed if the nurses did not know they were being observed. At the time of doing the research we felt that this outweighed any possible disregard of the rights of the staff to know they were being studied. The research site would be disguised in any publication of the results and neither nurses nor patients would be harmed. When the results were published the ward was disguised even to the extent that the observer's name had changed because she had subsequently married. I felt, and still feel, that no-one was harmed by our research on the surgical ward. However, Johnson argues that our technical and 'utilitarian' justification that the research was of general benefit ignored the human rights of the nurses we covertly studied, and that the use of deception by researchers raises important moral issues which we failed to address.

I think two lessons can be learned from my experience in doing this research. First, working alone can be difficult and unexpectedly 'dangerous' to oneself, and as a researcher you have a responsibility to look after yourself as well as attending to the people you are studying. One must be very sure and comfortable with the research methods one is using. In particular it is important to think through **all** aspects of the method: theoretical, methodological and ethical. One of the advantages of the unstructured interview for me is that it squares with my preference to be open and honest with people about what I am doing. Although covert research seemed a good idea at the time, I would now be very careful before using it as a method. I would still consider it, but the justifications for doing so would exercise me more greatly.

Second, it is very easy to succumb to the immediate pressures in the research environment and opt for pragmatic rather than theoretically and ethically well thought-out decisions. Researchers often complain about the necessity to get their health services research approved by ethical committees or other groups, but in retrospect the involvement of an ethical committee would have been helpful when we were considering the use of participant observation. It would have forced us to think more widely about our responsibilities to all the unwitting participants in the research. The involvement of such groups at the initial stages of the research process may help the researcher to clarify and resolve a number of potentially thorny practical and ethical issues associated with one's responsibility to one's subjects, such as: Who 'owns' the research? Who controls what is published and where it is published? What are the responsibilities of the researcher to his or her respondents? If there are conflicting views or interests, how are these to be dealt with? It is important to have someone who can provide support and advice, and if necessary act as a sounding board when things get difficult. It is also important to have continued advice and support. At the time of this research I was working largely on my own, with no adequate guidance or supervision in what were initially unfamiliar settings. My research meant that I was listening to sometimes very moving accounts and occasionally experiencing disturbing events (e.g. my first long chat with someone who wanted indirectly to discuss the fact that they were dying). In such circumstances it is easy to make simple errors because of one's involvement in the suffering of others. Not only is adequate support vital in such circumstances but so is personal comfort with one's research methods. Because I was comfortable in my choice of method and confident in its use I was able to deal with the pressures of evoking personal emotions in myself and others in what was initially a rather strange environment.

REFERENCES

Becker, H. S. (1967) Whose side are we on? *Social Problems* **14**, 239–247.

Cicourel, A. V. (1964) *Method and Measurement in Sociology*, Free Press, New York.

Denzin, N. (1989) *The Research Act: a Theoretical Discussion of Research Methods*, 3rd edn, Prentice Hall, Englewood Cliffs, NJ.

Field, D. (1984) 'We didn't want him to die on his own' – nurses' accounts of nursing dying patients. *Journal of Advanced Nursing* **9**, 59–70.

Field, D. (1989a) *Nursing the Dying*, Tavistock/Routledge, London.

Field, D. (1989b) Emotional involvement with the dying in a coronary care unit. *Nursing Times* **85**(2), 46–48.

Garfinkel, H. (1967) *Studies in Ethnomethodology*, Prentice Hall. Englewood Cliffs, NJ.

Glaser, B. G. & Strauss, A. L. (1965a) *Awareness of Dying*, Aldine, Chicago.

Glaser, B. G. & Strauss, A. L. (1965b) *Time for Dying*, Aldine, Chicago.

Glaser, B. G. & Strauss, A. L. (1968) *The Discovery of Grounded Theory: Strategies for Qualitative Research*, Aldine, Chicago.

Greenwald, H. P. & Nevitt, M. C. (1982) Physician attitudes towards communication with cancer patients. *Social Science & Medicine* **16**, 591–594.

Hammersley, M. & Atkinson, P. (1983) *Ethnography: Principles in Practice*, Tavistock, London.

Johnson, M. (1992) A silent conspiracy? Some ethical issues of participant observation in nursing research. *International Journal of Nursing Studies* **29**, 213–223.

Knight, M. & Field, D. (1981) A silent conspiracy: coping with dying cancer patients on an acute surgical ward. *Journal of Advanced Nursing* **6**, 221–229.

McIntosh, J. (1977) *Communication and Awareness in a Cancer Ward*, Croom Helm, London.

Mills, C. W. (1970) *The Sociological Imagination*, Pelican, Harmondsworth.

Oakley, A. (1981) Interviewing women: a contradiction in terms *Doing Feminist Research*, in H. Roberts (ed) Routledge & Kegan Paul, London, pp. 30–61.

Quint, J. C. (1968) *The Nurse and the Dying Patient*, Macmillan, New York.

Rubin, L. B. (1976) *Worlds of Pain: Life in the Working-Class Family*, Basic Books, New York.

Schwartz, H. & Jacobs, J. (1979) Qualitative Sociology: a Method to the Madness, Free Press, New York.

Sudnow, D. (1967) Passing on: the Social Organisation of Dying, Prentice Hall, Englewood Cliffs, NJ.

Tesch, R. (1990) Qualitative Analysis: Analysis Types and Software Tools, Falmer, London.

CHAPTER 9

Sensitive issues in sensitive settings: research in emergency departments

Beverley Raphael and Gwenneth Roberts

Research answering social health questions is often linked to sensitive and personal issues. Our aim in this chapter is to reflect on some of these political and ethical issues, issues that we have encountered in our own research practice. We will take for our particular examples of these complexities, our health research work in accident and emergency settings.

Some issues which are taken for granted by social science people are commonly considered problems by health workers. Some may appear as private or taboo in family or social settings, such as matters related to sexuality or death, e.g. childhood sexual abuse or domestic violence. Not only may there be perceptions which delineate these areas as 'private' or 'taboo' for enquiry, but there may also be considerable ambivalence in the broader society about the potential findings of such research. Furthermore, even the asking of relevant questions may be associated with the opening up of ambivalent, painful and traumatic experiences for the subjects participating, and hence a need for any research protocols to provide appropriate options and support in such instances. These matters aside, there is a common belief that questions about personal, sexual or intimate family relationships may cause problems. They are often perceived by those working in other research spheres (i.e. other than the social sciences) as potentially damaging on the one hand, or alternatively pointless on the other, because they are not associated with 'hard' findings such as biochemical test abnormalities.

Another issue of relevance is the nature of the health care setting in which social research questions may be asked. For instance, there may be perceptions of 'ownership' of the health care settings by particular professional interests in terms of meeting the needs of people. This is exemplified in the mental health care setting, where there may be acceptance if social research is seen to be answering questions identified as significant by that system. Alternatively, a surgical care unit may not see social research as answering questions to which it gives priority. In many instances the time and processes given to addressing the research may be seen as interfering with the purposes of the unit, or creating additional, and often by inference 'unnecessary', demands on staff and/or patients or clients.

Thus research aimed at examining particular social issues in relation to health, especially if concerning matters perceived as sensitive, or carried out in health care settings, may require complex negotiation which is well attuned to the politics of the systems involved. There is of course much to be said for working with these systems to frame research questions before developing a formal protocol, so that the research is relevant to, and owned by, all those involved.

When, as well as the factors identified above, there is an extra dimension to these problems, as for example in emergency health care provision, a complex and even more sensitive set of variables must be taken into account. Two research examples reflect this: disaster research and research in emergency medical settings such as emergency departments. The starting point for research questions, and even protocols, may be established beforehand with respect to these areas (Raphael et al., 1989; Singh et al., 1987) but the negotiation of entry may rely on the priorities given by those in charge of the 'life and death' problems handled in such environments.

The culture and practicalities of disasters are likely to demand triage of the injured, burial of the deceased, the provision of shelter, and other priorities of survival. It is extremely unlikely, even with carefully negotiated entry built on pre-existing conditions of mutual trust and collaboration, that it will be possible for social researchers to gain entry in the first post-emergency week. Thus the vast body of data covering social research on disasters provides little information on immediate response, except that gathered retrospectively. In some instances those involved in the provision of support have been able to contribute their observations (Valent, 1984) and this valuable qualitative material has added substantially to findings systematically gathered in close time frame (Weisaeth, 1985) covering the initial days or weeks. It has rarely been possible to work from pre-existing databases, but where this has been possible assessment has been made of the effects of acute experience in relation to basic attributes. Examples of these are demographic, social or personality characteristics which may have been present before the disaster and contributed either to reaction to the disaster or to the consequences that followed. As social research questions have gained priority, and the contributions of mental health professionals and other clinicians have been increasingly recognized, a more supportive framework has developed. Nevertheless, those affected by disaster must be protected not only from the convergence of well-meaning helpers, but also from the convergence of researchers. And the ethical questions also need to be addressed: the value of the research and its scientific validity must be taken into account. An emergency setting, even though often more appropriately addressed in naturalistic models of research, is no excuse for 'quick and dirty' projects that may make little contribution to those affected and may only add to the researcher's curriculum vitae.

Both the provision of the personal and social aspects of emergency health care to those affected by disasters and the exploration of social research questions must encompass the meeting of needs for those affected. This may be through participant research or alongside the provision of support, practical assistance or whatever is relevant. It is clear that the research to be carried out at the time of the emergency, rather than subsequently and retrospectively, must negotiate and fit with the emergency organization which develops. It will also need to fit with the culture of emergency services, including emergency health care providers. This question of fit may be critical, because there may be issues of life, death and survival that must take priority, where the social researcher may be seen as intrusive unless he or she has skills to also meet such needs. Furthermore, findings may be seen as potentially critical of the work done or its outcomes, and thus be threatening.

A number of social researchers, particularly mental health professionals, have been seen as contributing in ways that are important both in the actual emergency and in the period that follows, and in this way have been able to negotiate a place for research. For instance, Weisaeth (1985, 1989), a psychiatrist, studied a paint factory plant explosion in a workplace health model and was able to be involved shortly after the disaster. He was able to commence the development of a research study of behaviours during the traumatic event as described shortly afterwards, as well as anxiety and other reactions to the event. This study provided the first systematic description, admittedly retrospective, but close to the event of people's memories of their own behaviour and other people's descriptions of it. By providing for the psychological needs of those affected, many of whom required some counselling, he set up opportunities for data gathering which lasted through subsequent days, weeks and even years. This highlights the issue that is relevant in all such research but may be especially so for those working in emergency health care settings, i.e. the intervention effect of the research process. This may be accidental or deliberate, but even if unintentional should be taken into account. It may also be likely that people in such settings are in some sort of state of crisis (psychologically) and are more open to and affected by interactions with them, with the potential for positive or negative outcomes.

Thus there are a number of core themes with respect to research in emergency health care settings associated with disaster. These are: negotiated entry; negotiated research questions and protocols to answer these;

fitting with emergency organizations and systems and with priorities of survival and safety; recognizing and taking account of intervention aspects of the research; the principle of causing no harm.

These themes sit on the considerations of other social health research issues. These are: dealing with private or taboo matters; perceptions of the value and validity of social research; collaboration for research development to meet the needs of both parties; respect for the 'ownership' of the health care setting in which the research is to be carried out and in particular 'ownership' by the subjects of the research. These people may otherwise perceive the research as further control by the health system, and thus an additional source of disempowerment.

These themes are further highlighted when considering research in settings such as the emergency department of a major public hospital. Two such research projects will be discussed in this context.

PSYCHOSOCIAL MORBIDITY AND PREVENTIVE INTERVENTION

A project conducted at an emergency department (Singh *et al.*, 1987) aimed to examine levels of psychosocial morbidity and to provide crisis intervention for those found to be at high risk, or where indications suggested such morbidity was present. The department carrying out the research, the Department of Psychiatry, was already well established in the hospital and known to staff through its consultation–liaison service, which provided psychiatric assessment and guidance for the care of patients in general medical and surgical settings. Thus the researchers were known and trusted by the health care system and had previously been seen in helpful roles in the section that was to be the research focus. Previous research in the USA had established the high levels of psychosocial morbidity in such settings but no equivalent research had been carried out in Australia. Negotiations took place with the emergency department and it was agreed that these matters were significant and of concern to this extremely busy unit. Anxieties about the potential intrusiveness of the project – that it might 'get in the way', or interfere with emergency management, particularly at times of crisis – were discussed. The need for the research to be non-intrusive and part of normal routine was emphasized. The problems of where to place the research assistant, where he or she would fit in space which was at a premium, and where the person who would provide crisis intervention would be located, were all seen as significant issues. The protocol required a brief screening questionnaire to detect risk factors (stressful life events, attachments and support) and levels of distress or disorder (Goldberg 1972). This was to be scored by a research assistant on the spot and then those meeting high-risk criteria would be randomly allocated to intervention with a skilled and empathic clinical psychologist, with follow-up assessment of intervention and control groups six months later.

The emergency department and the research group worked with these questions at some length. A solution which met the needs of both sides was the appointment to this project of a senior general nurse who also had research assistant experience. The nurse researcher had trained at this hospital, was well known to staff, familiar with the emergency system and skilled in questionnaire administration. It was also agreed that he/she would wear a uniform to fit in further. This project worked extremely well in its screening phase, with the research nurse being seen as highly acceptable to the emergency department and viewed very positively by patients. However, fitting so well brought a further complication – and perhaps a 'finding' that links to findings in the disaster area. Having been empathically assessed and screened by someone clearly identified as part of the hospital system, the vast majority of people at risk were unwilling to take the next step to a counsellor. Even though mechanisms of referral were somewhat similar to those for further assessment in other spheres, they could not, of course, be prescribed or directed in the way that referrals to specialists or tests were made, nor with the same power and authority that was part of the emergency care ethos. Whether patients subtly realized this, or their needs were seen as already being met by the screening process was unclear, although the general feeling was that the latter applied. Thus this project was successful in fitting into the emergency care setting and established some significant findings (the probable prevalence of minor psychiatric morbidity in adults presenting to the emergency department was estimated at 27%). However, we were unable to answer our central research question about the effectiveness or otherwise of crisis intervention in diminishing psychosocial morbidity and improving outcomes for those presenting in such settings.

DOMESTIC VIOLENCE PRESENTATIONS AND DETECTION

This study was developed to examine the presentation of patients with domestic violence problems at a large emergency department, to assess whether this aspect was appropriately detected and dealt with and, if not, whether interventions including the education of medical and nursing staff would enhance outcomes (Roberts *et al.*, 1993b). Funding for this project was provided by the Queensland Department of Family Services and Aboriginal and Islander Affairs, the Criminology Research Council and Queensland Health. The project engendered many issues of sensitivity. Domestic violence is frequently seen as a taboo and private family affair where intrusion should not take place. There are potential risks to clients and possibly even staff associated with detection. How such assessment fits with the triage urgency and time requirements of this high-intensity unit is also important. The potential for negative findings that could be critical of staff functioning, e.g. failure to detect victims, was also a concern. Other issues which created dilemmas were: poor medical records; what to do with those detected; how to deal with those in acute need in terms of safety, survival or mental health; the value and validity of this 'soft' research; the likelihood of education enhancing the effectiveness of staff actions; and the possible 'harmful' effects of the research.

The climate of negotiation for research entry was helped by a number of factors. Among the most important of these were: a state government report highlighting the high level of domestic violence in the community; a national agenda addressing violence against women; US data reporting significant levels of presentation in this setting; and a sympathetic director of the emergency service who agreed with the importance of the issue.

Negotiations for the final research protocol were able to be carried out after a pilot study by the research officer for this project. Here, too, acceptability of the person in this system was facilitated by the fact that the appointee was a senior nurse with a qualification in psychology. Thus the entry of the worker was easily achieved because of her knowledge of such systems and her capacity to engage them, their structures, language and functioning. The screening instrument which evolved after initial testing had to be particularly brief and systems of referral for those at risk identified. Furthermore, these negotiations had to encompass all levels of staff, to ensure acceptability throughout the system, and to cover the opening hours of the department, e.g. through night and evening shifts. Initially we hoped that the screening measure could be given out and collected by the nursing staff working in the system, but this proved to be ineffective during the pilot study.

Our negotiations with medical staff revealed a number of concerns that had to be worked through. There appeared to be some reluctance among doctors to be involved in this part of the patient's assessment or history taking. There was concern about whether questionnaires about domestic violence, if administered before the patient's medical assessment, would affect their emotional state in relation to the assessment. There was concern that the patients would be threatened or offended by being asked these questions, or upset and disturbed by them. There was a general belief that domestic violence was not frequent and not relevant to the emergency department. These concerns were addressed so that the final research protocol was accepted. Nursing staff had few concerns about the research process and gave support to the protocols.

Screening of people presenting to the emergency department was then set in place, with the senior research officer and research assistants all experienced in the emergency care environment and domestic violence doing the interviewing. Thus two successful prevalence studies were carried out, one before as a baseline measure, and one after an educational intervention. These studies were linked to two case-control studies, examining detection rates in patient records during both 12-month periods preceding the prevalence studies. Further analysis identified those variables that differentiated cases and controls. The medical records examination was carried out by a senior and respected psychiatrist, also well known in the hospital setting. The differential rates of detection in the two case-control studies aimed to measure the outcome of the educational intervention.

As with the previous study, we originally intended that the effectiveness of intervention with those patients detected by this screening would be assessed in a randomized controlled trial. A personal trauma clinic was set up alongside other clinics to which people were referred from the emergency department. We intended that this clinic should also serve as a referral point for victims of domestic violence and other psychologically traumatic experiences, but not one person screened and referred in this initial setting was prepared to go to this service for follow-up. Thus the initial part of the study proved the impossibility of this part of the research project, perhaps highlighting the 'all-in-one' need of those who present. As an aside, it is of interest to note that despite extensive publicity about the nature of this clinic and its role, and proclaimed need in this area, referrals were few and often inappropriate.

The initial screening phase was successful and showed that 23% of women and 6% of men had a history of domestic violence in their lifetime, and that every 50th woman presenting to the emergency department had domestic violence injuries or problems. During this period the social work department provided emergency response to those detected and in acute need, and thus the intervention effect became focused on this service. However, this could not be assessed for outcome or incorporated as a randomized controlled trial. It should also be noted that the findings of the research and the requirements through recognition of this problem, both in the broader community and increasingly in the hospital setting, led to the establishment of an after-hours social work service. This evolved to deal with these and other problems which we found had presented most frequently in the night and in the latter part of the week, often in line with pay day and associated heavy male drinking patterns on Fridays and Saturdays of each week and public holidays. Thus an unintended but needed intervention evolved from this research, but could not be evaluated in the research process.

The initial phase of the study revealed relatively low detection rates of domestic violence – 31% of those who self-reported domestic violence within the last week and 6.4% of those with a lifetime history were recorded. The educational intervention aimed at enhancing this detection rate, and hopefully appropriate actions, then had to be devised to fit with the emergency medical care settings and the culture and ethos of this system. The educational programme was conducted after a baseline survey of knowledge and attitudes in this area, covering medical and nursing staff. It aimed to deal with necessary knowledge and attitude change. An identical survey was carried out after the education programme to measure the process and impact evaluation of the educational intervention.

In formulating the education programme, expertise was sought from a senior social worker and others who had been involved in this field and carried out education. Consultations were held with the medical and nursing directors as to the most appropriate formats and protocols. It should be noted that at the same time the state health department produced a protocol on domestic violence, presented in the form of a poster to be distributed to Queensland hospitals, and the poster was evaluated in this study. Problems identified were the need to make this programme and its information fit with the time urgency, and life and death priorities, of this setting. To respond to this a pocket card was developed for medical and nursing staff with a format similar to that used in emergency resuscitation care. This material, with posters and other literature about domestic violence, combined with presentations by police, social workers and the senior research officer, and case presentations by the senior psychiatrist in the hospital, constituted the education programme, which was repeated for relevant groups throughout the intervention period.

The results of attendance and participation in the education programme, plus its effects on knowledge and attitudes, showed some positive impact. This was more successful on the whole for nurses rather than doctors, as their attendance was better and less likely to be interrupted by urgent paging for other emergency tasks. Rapid turnover of resident medical officers also proved a significant problem when attempting to assess any outcomes (questionnaire response rates were low), for they were unlikely to be still in the emergency department at the time of the second knowledge and attitudes survey. Questionnaires were often mailed to them at provincial or rural hospitals during the period when the second case-control study was carried out.

After completion of the study programme, educational materials were left with senior staff in the emergency department for the purpose of training the staff who would be working in the department during the period of testing detection rates in the second case-control study. The effectiveness of different parts of the educational programme was assessed and one of the most successful parts was the pocket card (Roberts *et al.*, 1993a). Thus while the shaping of the programme to fit the needs of the system was to some degree effective, as demonstrated in the research results, at least in terms of skills, knowledge and attitudes, it could not fit adequately with the culture of rapid change, urgent demands and rapid response.

Outcome evaluation revealed little change in overall detection rates, perhaps reflecting the difficulties of saturating the system and reaching the relevant people in the educational intervention, or the limitations of its effectiveness as a relatively brief measure. In the second prevalence study results showed that half of those presenting directly as a result of domestic violence were detected, highlighting the need for much further work in this sphere. Although overall detection rates did not change, there was a constant number of referrals to the after-hours social work service which had been instituted. However, the research team was unable to evaluate this service.

Thus the project and education programme became accepted and incorporated into the system while it ran, and had some lasting effects in terms of intervention in the broadest sense: the after-hours social work service; the pocket card; modification of the posters and protocols; and incorporation of educational input into the resident medical officers' handbook and emergency department manual. Materials formulated for this project were subsequently used in domestic violence training programmes for medical and nursing staff in Queensland public hospitals. Further research in this field has also been carried out in other centres using similar methods.

We noted above that one of the ethical constraints that is critical to any research is 'first to do no harm'. There were no reports indicating that the opening up of these questions had proved to be unduly stressful for the patients who participated, or had created additional difficulties for the staff involved. Response rates to the screening questionnaire were high and many patients indicated that they felt positively about the research. Nevertheless, there were many horrendous circumstances which highlight the difficulties and risks. Sometimes it was a problem to assess or interview a victim of domestic violence in a private or secure setting away from a partner who was a potential or actual abuser. Issues of privacy and anonymity were a source of stress: for instance, one woman had escaped an abusive husband in one state of Australia and brought her children with her, with a changed name and a new address. A welfare clerk had given her husband her name and address and she presented with severe battering, which had resulted when he found her. Another woman who had to be admitted was pursued by her husband into the ward, where he made further life-threatening attacks, even endangering ward and security staff.

This work proved to be very stressful for research staff and all involved. Not only was there identification with the victim's traumatization, but often the sense of helplessness that little could be done. Experience by research staff working in such areas is a significant factor. This was even more the case in this setting, because the research workers were women and most of the victims were women, reinforcing identification. It should also be remembered that there are high rates of sexual and physical abuse and domestic violence in the community and it is highly likely that some workers themselves may have had similar experiences. Thus the stress issue must be recognized and appropriate review, supervision and debriefing processes set in place, to prevent burnout, support the worker and, from the research point of view, to ensure that such factors do not interfere adversely with the research process. These matters need to be taken into account in research staff selection and training, as well as protocol development.

Another issue of concern to health professionals is that the topic of domestic violence is sometimes viewed naively as 'a feminist takeover', as expressed by one health professional. While it must be acknowledged that the feminist movement has played a major part in placing this topic on the public agenda (Schechter, 1982), the high rate of presentation of victims of domestic violence at the emergency department highlights the need for health care systems to take this problem seriously on its own terms.

ETHICS IN EMERGENCY HEALTH CARE RESEARCH

As can be seen from the above there are many ethical issues, both those that relate to impact on systems of care as well as those directly affecting subjects and workers. They need to be carefully taken into account and dealt with at every stage, from the negotiations of collaboration and research questions to the elucidation of research methods. It is clear that the realities of life and death urgency and priorities in such settings must be taken into account and should not be denied by researchers with other priorities. Nevertheless, the culture of emergency care may deny the realities of social aspects of health, and the culture may proclaim more urgency upon this than reality substantiates. This is clear from the continuing evidence of high levels of psychosocial presentation in emergency departments, which often function in or near primary care models. There is a need for both cultures to adapt.

A further issue is the research method chosen and its ethical and professional acceptance in such settings. Emergency health care operates in factual, hard, urgent, scientific and technical models. Research may require similar or different frameworks, but the processes of the health care system and the realities of those presenting may mean that the protocols proposed cannot be carried through, at least to their full extent. Furthermore, qualitative methods such as ethnographic studies may have much to offer, especially if linked to other data that are quantitative. Yet it may be difficult for those in charge of access, and the scientific and ethics committees reviewing protocols, to accept these 'softer' methodological contributions. Coincidental observations have been made which might have been better covered by such methods. Such observations include patients overhearing staff make negative comments about them and any psychological or social problems they had (they were described as 'wasting time', 'manipulative', 'seductive', 'bludging', 'histrionic', 'no good' or 'enjoying it'); and staff avoiding or giving short shrift to those with sensitive or psychosocial problems. These matters need to be addressed in research, but of course also much more basically in health care worker education. They might more easily and more effectively be addressed if technical negotiations about research priorities address or are able to complement the clinical priorities of providers in these settings.

There are many unanswered and important questions with respect to emergency health care, in places such as emergency departments and also in intensive care, medical evacuation and response teams, and so forth. These questions cover matters such as decisions to resuscitate or discontinue life support; how the highly sensitive matter of requests for organ donation are handled with shocked and acutely bereaved family members; whether to save or not to save extremely premature infants; how informed consent is gained in emergency situations; and what are stressor effects on health care staff. It would be appropriate for emergency health care providers and social researchers to identify and work together to achieve optimal processes or protocols to answer these and many other critical questions.

REFERENCES

Goldberg, D.P. (1972) *The Detection of Psychiatric Illness by Questionnaire*, Oxford University Press, Oxford.

Raphael, B., Lundin, T. and Weisaeth, L. (1989) A research method for the study of psychological and psychiatric aspects of disaster. *Acta Psychiatrica Scandinavica* **80**, Suppl. 353, 1–75.

Roberts, G., Lawrence, J., Raphael, B. *et al.* (1993a) Domestic violence and health professionals. Letter to the Editor. *Medical Journal of Australia* **158**, 861.

Roberts, G., O'Toole, B., Lawrence, J. and Raphael, B. (1993b) Domestic violence in a hospital emergency department. *Medical Journal of Australia* **159**, 307–10.

Schechter, S. (1982) *Women and Male Violence*, South End Press, Boston.

Singh, B., Lewin, T., Raphael, B. *et al.* (1987) Minor psychiatric morbidity in a casualty population: identification, attempted intervention and six-month follow-up. *Australian and New Zealand Journal of Psychiatry* **21**, 231–40.

Valent, P. (1984) The Ash Wednesday bush fires. *Medical Journal of Australia* **141**, 291–300.

Weisaeth, L. (1985) Post-traumatic stress disorder after an industrial disaster: prevalences, etiological and prognostic factors, in *Psychiatry – the State of the Art*, eds P.Pichot, P.Berner, R.Wolf and K.Thau, Plenum Press, New York, pp. 299–307.

Weisaeth, L. (1989) The stressors and the post-traumatic stress syndrome after an industrial disaster. *Acta Psychiatrica Scandinavica* **80**, Suppl. 355, 25–37.

CHAPTER 10

Birth as euphoria: the social meaning of birth

Karen Lane

INTRODUCTION

This chapter addresses the problem of the normative nature of scientific assumptions and associated methodologies related to birthing. The argument will draw upon comparative policy frameworks in Britain and Australia, it will examine the philosophical underpinnings related to birthing policies in each country, and it will review the macrostatistical data related to institutional regimes and birthing practices.

British and Australian policy documents released over the last 2 years have critically addressed postwar birthing regimes and practices. Recommended changes have promoted a greater role for GPs and midwives, an expanded set of options for women and a plurality of models of care for the low-risk women who constitute the majority of maternity cases. Significantly, the documents have been very critical of obstetric practices, especially routine interventions for which no reliable evaluations existed prior to use. Current assessment insists that interventions have not reduced mortality rates, and in some cases they are considered to carry more risks than those they are designed to avoid. Henceforth all routine obstetric interventions are to be evaluated by randomized control trials (Winterton Committee, 1992; NHMRC, 1994).

The World Health Organization, at a meeting in Fortaleza, Brazil (1994), endorsed this view. These interventions included amniotomy (artificial breaking of fetal membranes); pharmacological induction of labour; adoption of the lithotomy position in delivery or labour (still practised in eastern Europe but losing favour in western Europe, the United States and Australia); drugs for pain relief, including epidural, unless specifically required to prevent a complication; routine intrapartum electronic fetal monitoring; and episiotomy. The meeting agreed that caesarean section, forceps and vacuum extraction rates were unaccountably high. It was also alarming that the highest rates were recorded in countries with large numbers of obstetricians in private practice caring for normal pregnant and birthing women (Marsden, 1994).

As a result of these kinds of critiques, birthing policy in advanced liberal democracies is beginning to demonstrate two distinct policy frameworks. Holland and, more recently, Britain have to some extent departed from a medical model of birthing. It is more accurate to describe the arrangements in those countries as a bifurcated model. This means that the medical model of birthing, while still dominant, shows signs of attenuation towards a more woman-centred view.

An undiluted medical model is more characteristic of Australian practices. Although obstetric control has come under fire in Australia, proposed arrangements will not seriously dislodge medical dominance, which rests partially on findings drawn from quantitative survey questionnaires about levels of satisfaction with existing arrangements. This chapter argues that quantitative methodologies are inadequate tools to access the contradictions and complexities of womens' experiences of birthing. Thus, the survey findings have provided an entirely inadequate basis for constructing a universal maternity system. The complacency with existing arrangements is demonstrated in constrained options for women concerning choice of location and type of maternity care. These arguments are explored in a comparative analysis of birthing policies and philosophies in Britain and Australia.

TWO PHILOSOPHICAL VIEWS OF CHILDBIRTH

A woman-centred view of birthing, or a social model, may be summed up by the following philosophy:

> Becoming a mother is not an illness. It is not an abnormality. It is a normal process which occurs during the lives of the majority of women and can indeed be seen as a manifestation of health. It is physically very demanding and is a time when women are vulnerable in many ways. They require help and support during the process of being pregnant, giving birth, and postnatally and some of this, though not all, needs professional help. In some circumstances the quality of the professional help is literally vital. But it is the mother who gives birth and it is she who will have the lifelong commitment which motherhood brings. She is the most active participant in the birth process. Her interests are intimately bound up with those of her baby. (Winterton Committee, 1992)

This view sees the body as a complex whole. It understands that emotional and physical aspects of human life cannot be divorced from each other and that the social context of birthing (including the social history of the mother, her perception of social and power relations within the birthplace, and her sense of control) is a critical and determinant feature of the birthing process. This view reintroduces the mother as the agent and centralizes the mother/child relationship. According to the social model, safety and emotional satisfaction cannot be divorced from each other, because emotional ease is a precondition for an unimpeded birth free from interventions, associated morbidities and possible mortality.

The orthodox obstetric view of childbirth is enscapsulated in the following comment made by a specialist obstetrician giving evidence to the Winterton Committee in 1992:

> There are low risk and high risk pregnancies, but there is not a no risk group. Because all are at risk, the delivery suite is an intensive care area and should be staffed as such, both to deal with emergencies and to monitor mother and fetus in labour to prevent serious problems. More use of fetal scalp sampling should be encouraged.

Further, he commented that 'analgesia is required in almost all labours' (Winterton Committee, 1992). In 1989, the President of RACOG Australia, Dr J. O'Loughlin, indicated support for this view by saying that 'Nature is a lousy midwife'. A vitriolic rejoinder rapidly emanated from members of the Australian College of Midwives, who replied that 'Nature could equally be a lousy obstetrician' (Bundy, 1993).

The medical view of birthing sees the body as essentially pathological. It divorces emotional and contextual factors from the physical and reifies risk. The philosophy derives from the positivistic philosophy of Descartes, who inserted an irreconcilable division between the mind, or emotions, and the body. Within this framework, the centrality of experience, feeling, emotion and the interpretation by individuals of their social and physical world is negated (Turner, 1987). When extrapolated to birthing, Cartesian philosophy (and medical theory) understands childbirth as a set of discrete physical, chemical and muscular changes. A medical view imposes precise limits on each of the stages in abstraction from the emotional and social context in which those changes take place, and which may have significantly caused the physiological changes (or, in the case of 'delay in progress', non-changes). Birthing ceases to be a social and cultural event. Under this view, the main relationship occurs between the doctor and the baby. The doctor neutralizes the agency of the mother by the use of scientific apparatus to monitor the baby, to augment its passage and finally perhaps to extract it from the mother's body.

As the above statement indicates, medical personnel conceptualize birthing as a purely physiological process where emotional and interpretive factors are denied explanatory and causal power. Since the overriding concern of obstetricians is the prior detection of any precipitous and unexpected events, modern obstetrics has become characterized by an obsessive definition of what is 'normal'. There has been a tendency to redefine what is normal by imposing progressively constrained parameters.

Only women of a certain age, parity and medical history will be defined as normal. Conversely, the recategorization of what is abnormal and the community of those at risk has expanded accordingly (Chalmers, 1978). A major consequence has been the designation of all birthing mothers as a community at risk, although some may be at more risk than others. This pathologizing of all maternity cases has led to the aphorism that a safe birth can only be assured in retrospect. Further, as Douglas (1990) has argued, the imposition of an aura of risk serves as a political weapon in the definition of those who are morally promiscuous because they dispute medical advice. The equation between risk and sinning is a useful concept in relation to birthing. It appears to be a common practice among medical personnel to cast those who shun hospitalization as being morally invidious.

The ostensibly unpredictable nature of the body during birthing has legitimized the use of multiphasic screening procedures designed not just to remedy but to pre-empt any departures from the normal before they actually occur. For example, each stage of labour and delivery is monitored and measured carefully with scientific apparatus. Any departure from what is regarded as normal change is met with intervention by medical professionals to ensure that the birth proceeds according to predetermined parameters. The phenomenon known as the 'cascade of intervention' is the logical outcome (World Health Organization, 1985; Department of Health, Victoria, 1990: NHMRC, 1994). However, these parameters are themselves constructed according to a pathological view of the body, according to which the most important measure of a successful birth is one where both the mother and the child remain alive. Maternal satisfaction and the quality of relations surrounding and preceding the birth remain substantially outside the medical ambit of concern, especially 6 weeks after the birth when medical reponsibility formally ceases.

The juxtaposition of these alternative views of birthing is examined in relation to policies in Britain and Australia.

MATERNITY SERVICES IN BRITAIN

In Britain, the UK Department of Health (Winterton Committee, 1992) eschewed the medical model of care which had achieved dominance after the National Health Service Act of 1946. This provided free maternity services under the care of GPs. Formerly, the majority of maternity services were provided by midwives at the local authority level. Their professional autonomy gradually became eroded in the postwar period as a consequence of successive government inquiries which endorsed a medical model of care and its corollary – the universal hospitalization of women (Oakley, 1986; Tew, 1990).

In 1992 the Winterton Committee recommendations represented a watershed in maternity services, shifting the emphasis from the medical model to a woman-centred model. Specifically, the report strongly criticized the current practice whereby 98% of women delivered in hospitals under shared-care arrangements with GP and obstetrician. Unequivocally, the report stated that 'hospitals are not the appropriate place to care for healthy women'. The recommendations emphasized that continuity of care and carer, increased access to information in the antenatal period to allow women to make informed choices about place of birth and carer, and a much expanded role for midwives should be put in place. Institutionally, these objectives were seen to be best served by the development of midwife-managed maternity units inside and outside hospitals, and the granting to midwives the right to admit women to public hospitals and to take full responsibility for the women under their care. In sum, the report endorsed the full professional status of midwives. It also recommended midwifery control over training procedures and the setting of professional standards. In summary, the Winterton Report substantially negated the legitimacy of interventionism and medical paternalism in relation to birthing women and to professional midwifery practice.

Home birth in Britain

Perhaps this challenge to medical paternalism is most cogently demonstrated in relation to the new British approach to home birth. The report noted that birthing at home or in a small maternity unit had been denied to women on the grounds of non-safety. It recommended that the option of giving birth in a small maternity unit (that is, one with low-level technology) or at home should be restored. GPs were directed to facilitate the wishes of women, especially in relation to choice of setting as well as midwife-only care, and they were not permitted to remove home-birth women from their lists (Winterton Committee, 1992). In the light of previous inquiries, which had substantiated the universal hospitalization of women and the denigration of home birth, this initiative must be seen as profoundly critical of orthodox obstetric practice. In Australia, exactly the reverse has applied.

MATERNITY SERVICES IN AUSTRALIA

In February 1994, the National Health and Medical Research Council of Australia published a draft report entitled *Options for Effective Care in Childbirth*. The report considered present maternity services and community pressures for change. It made special mention of the needs of migrant, Aboriginal and adolescent pregnant women. The document also aimed to promote new strategies for care in childbirth and postnatal care, for the training of midwives and obstetricians, for regional and emergency services and for data collection and research.

At first glance, the proposals offered a significant shift from a medical model of care. For example, the report documented 'an increasing desire [by consumers] for midwives to provide a greater input into maternity services' (NHMRC, 1994). It also proposed as a general basis for its recommendations an expanded range of options and models for maternity care. Of special note was the recognition that 'women's experiences and levels of satisfaction with different options of care should also be evaluated in randomized trials as a matter of priority'. The issue of maternal satisfaction is important. In the past obstetric science has stressed mortality or safety as the only indicators of a successful birth. In other words, until recent years an obstetrician would assess a successful birth as one where both the mother and child remained alive after the event. Trauma, satisfaction, depression and short- and longer-term morbidity arising out of medical procedures remained inert in the medical judgement of a good birth. By contrast, a progressive element of the report was the recognition that maternal satisfaction should be regarded as a decisive factor in the policy process.

Critique of existing practices

Like the WHO resolutions and the Winterton Report, the NHMRC report (1994) echoed a critique of the high levels of intervention in Australian hospitals. It noted that the caesarean section rate in Australia was among the highest in the world. Discussion documented the trend towards the increasing use of regional analgesia or epidural block rather than more simple methods (baths, massage and mobility), simply because staff had not been trained in more rudimentary and less invasive methods and because epidural block was readily available in many obstetric units. It noted that epidural analgesia may result in short-term pain relief but irremedial longer-term backache. The report noted the admirable decline in the use of oxytocic agents to accelerate labour. A 'wait and see' approach had shown a deceleration of the fetal heart rate and hence less need for intervention for fetal distress. Further, the almost universal adoption of electronic fetal monitoring was seen to offer only a marginal benefit to the fetus in terms of reduced number of neonatal convulsions and more importantly, no reduction in the incidence of cerebral palsy for which the test was routinely employed. The authors of the report agreed that cardiotocography provided only interim information about the health of the fetus and that inter- and intra-observer errors in the interpretation of fetal heart rate recordings were common. Overall, the report admonished the use of routine measurement and observation techniques on the grounds that they had been utilized more often on the basis of myth and fashion than carefully planned and scientific evaluation. In summary, the authors recommended that 'Whenever possible an assessment of the value of any intervention should be judged by evidence from randomized trials' (NHMRC, 1994).

These are radical and refreshing critiques of commonplace obstetric practices. Yet the proposed arrangements failed to fully extend the options and models of care available to mothers, despite a stated intention of the Council to do so. The policy makers obviously believed that birthing centres within major maternity hospitals would expand options for women and that the new arrangements would offer safety, control over the birthing process by mothers, access to and sharing of information and continuity of care (NHMRC, 1994). Without a doubt, the shift to birthing centres from labour wards will be a significant advance on present arrangements, where 98% of women deliver their babies in high-technology maternity units in hospitals and where intervention is commonplace and extensive, as noted above. It is the case that free-standing birthing centres generally offer a discernible departure from hospital régimes because they encourage control by women, they provide continuity of care from one professional, free mobility during labour and a non-interventionist birthing philosophy. However – and this is centrally important – the Panel overtly discredited the idea of free-standing birthing centres, that is, birthing centres remote from a maternity unit and staffed entirely by midwives. In other words, the dominant model of care will remain the medical model because birthing centres within maternity hospitals remain under general obstetric control. Thus, integrated birthing centres do not depart significantly from medical model philosophies. This argument is illustrated by analysing data from studies of integrated birthing centres in Australia.

Integrated Birthing Centres

Birthing units located within tertiary maternity centres are highly cautious in their selection of what they regard as low-risk women. Only women with no previous medical, gynaecological or obstetric history are included. Age and parity (the number of previous births) are also determining factors. Selection based on this set of criteria effectively excludes large numbers of women. A subsequent culling occurs at later stages.

Another way of illustrating this point is to cite the transfer rates from birthing centre to obstetric ward. In a study by Permezel *et al.* (1987) of 1794 low-risk women selected for delivery in the birthing unit of the Royal Women's Hospital, Melbourne, only 68.4% remained to deliver there. In other words, the transfer rate was 34.4%. In other studies, Klein *et al.* (1983) found that 48% of nulliparous women were transferred and 25% of multiparous women were transferred from a GPU unit to an obstetric ward. Morris *et al.* (1986) found that 37.6% were transferred; Linder Pelz *et al.* (1990) found that 30% transferred from birthing centre to labour ward.

By contrast, the transfer rate from home to hospital in Australia in 1990 was 12.9% (44% of these transferred because of lack of progress; Bastian and Lancaster, 1990). Similarly, Woodcock *et al.* (1990) reported a lower transfer rate from home to hospital of 24.6%. Crotty *et al.* (1990) reported a 17% transfer rate. In summary, the initial assessment for entry to birthing centres will exclude significant numbers of women. Subsequent culling will again occur at later stages.

Permezel *et al.* (1987) reported, for example, that a total of 50% of women were excluded from the birthing unit at the Royal Women's Hospital, Melbourne: 18% were initially deemed ineligible, and a further 32% were transferred out either during labour or after delivery. Permezel *et al.* (1987) concluded that these figures not only rendered home birth a hazardous option, but that 'despite careful selection of a low-risk population there remains a persistent incidence of potential serious complications and a continuing need for obstetric intervention'. This conclusion was affirmed by Linder-Pelz *et al.* (1990) as a result of a study of the Royal Hospital for Women, Sydney. In comparing the birthing centre entrants with women who gave birth in the labour ward and with those who transferred from birthing centre to labour ward in the intrapartum period, the authors concluded that:

> ...we have limited ability to predict which pregnancies will have complications. [Therefore].. there is a need for birth centres to have adequate and appropriate medical back-up regardless of how favourable the assessed prenatal risk is.

It is argued here that most transfers from birthing centre to labour ward occur on spurious medical grounds. In the Linder-Pelz study, for example, 90% of the interventions and transfers occurred because of dysfunctional labour, secondary arrest of dilatation, syntocinon augmentation and elective induction (including epidural, operative forceps, outlet forceps and caesarean section). In the Linder-Pelz study no more than 17% occurred for what are considered serious obstetric conditions, such as pre-eclampsia (3%) or premature rupture of membranes (13.9%). It is salient to note from a sociological perspective that the conditions attributed to the 90% who transferred are not causes, but descriptions of states of being. Failure to progress, or delay in progress (as these conditions are sometimes known), can be attributed to women's negative perceptions of their physical and social environment. Mention should also be made of the 45.4% of Victorian women birthing in hospitals in 1988 who required either induction, augmentation or elective caesarean section as a result of 'failure to progress' (Department of Health, Victoria, 1990).

Medical theory remains satisfied that the majority of women have a dysfunctional anatomy because a medical view of the body is built on the assumption of essential pathology. However, if the body is seen as non-pathological, and if birthing is seen as a social and cultural event, then the causes of failure to progress must be sought in the conditions surrounding the birth.

In my qualitative study of women's birthing experiences,[1] women who failed to progress reported that they had experienced degrees of stress related to negative social relations in their environment. This kind of negativity may also be experienced at home but, as the statistics for transfer from birthing centre to labour ward show, the stress is more likely to be experienced in hospital. Reports from women affirm that negative relations with hospital staff or fear of the hospital or its accoutrements may either cause considerable anxiety and/or delay in the birthing process. Maternal distress is common because pregnant women and women in labour have already assumed a protective role in relation to their baby. They are thus unusually alert to environmental conditions. Any positive or negative factors in interaction or procedure assume exaggerated proportions. For example, women often remark that they became upset because of offhand or critical comments made by hospital staff. And many 'good' labours cease on hospital admission. It is logical to assume that a condition which continues to afflict around 50% of labouring women would attract attention from medical researchers. Yet medical theory remains inert to such a phenomenon because it blindly accepts the pathology of the body (and especially women's bodies) as the ontological grounding of medical practice. Significantly, there are no medical studies of delayed labour, but a proliferation of studies of the exact dosage of labour stimulants.

The 3% of women suffering from pre-eclampsia (high blood pressure) in the Linder-Pelz *et al.* (1990) study, who were also included in the transferred cohort, may arguably have experienced similar anxieties about their environment. Such arguments and studies have not been documented, for the reasons outlined above. However, one independent midwife offered an example of such a case which, she asserts, is not unexpected. This particular mother had reported a rapid rise in blood pressure readings when a particular staff member administered the procedure. This did not occur after the midwife had tutored the mother in positive visualization techniques.

A major medical reason for transfer in the Linder-Pelz study was attributed to premature rupture of membranes (13.9% of women in the study). From a sociological perspective this is a highly questionable basis for

---

1   The study comprised 40 women in total. Twenty women were interviewed in Britain and 20 in Australia (10 who delivered at home and 10 who delivered in hospital in each case). It was often the case that the home-birth women had previously given birth in hospital. The British respondents had attended independent childbirth educators (classes run by the NCT). In Australia respondents had attended either a local community health centre for their education or they had attended the hospital at which they delivered their baby. The interviews were designed to find out what women desired from a 'good birth', and whether there were differences or similarities among hospital and home-birth women. The interviews were conducted between 1992 and 1994.

transfer. The orthodox obstetric view is that premature rupture of the membranes is a serious medical condition because of the possibility of infection and subsequent death of the fetus. However, there is no medical study to support this assumption: it is merely one of those procedures identified by the NHMRC report as based more upon myth and fashion than accredited inquiry. In summary, all of the conditions cited as reasons for transfer and, therefore, for ruling out free-standing birthing centres and home birth, may be regarded as spurious from the point of view of a social model of birthing. Of course, there are solid reasons from a medical point of view. However, a social model of birthing may easily render these grounds as evidence of the importance of emotional equilibrium, predictability, familiarity and continuity of carer(s).

Free-standing birthing centres

There are very few free-standing birthing centres which can be compared with integrated centres in terms of intervention rates and mortality rates. However, the one such experimental centre in Victoria, the Moorabin Birth Centre, which is staffed entirely by midwives under a non-interventionist model of care, shows comparatively low intervention rates and a low perinatal mortality rate (1.3/100 compared with the national PNMR of 3.5/1000) (Biro and Lumley, 1991). Statistics for 1993 show that transfers before labour were 14.3% and transfers during labour were only 10.5%. Again, most of the intrapartum transfers (43 out of 62) were attributed to rupture of membranes, delay in progress or need for pain relief (epidural). Similarly, the Boothville Maternity Hospital's free-standing birthing centre in Brisbane reported a 4.9/1000 perinatal mortality rate (including transferred cases), a low intervention rate (7.1%% forceps delivery and 9.3% caesarean section rate), a low narcotic analgesia rate (12%) and a minimal transfer rate to larger centres (2.8% for mother and baby) over a 14-year period. Notably, the centre offers continuity of care, tactile and vocal analgesia (as opposed to chemical pain relief), freedom to choose delivery position, and a 'gentle birth' method of delivery for the baby (Elliott, 1992).

The point being argued here is that integrated birthing centres within tertiary maternity units (those housing high-technology and emergency facilities) as opposed to independent birthing centres, do not necessarily offer women a greatly expanded set of choices. This is particularly the case when obstetric guidelines determine the selection criteria and when many of the criteria for exclusion (discussed above) are highly questionable.

Integrated birthing units may also prove to be non-expansive when midwifery care is placed under obstetric guidelines. This is because the question of expanded models is not simply a question of location, but also of the philosophy of care. Midwives in Australia who first train as nurses are more likely to regard themselves are obstetric assistants. Birthing centres tacitly controlled by obstetric staff employed by the hospital encourage a deprofessionalized role for midwives. Indeed, the professional subordination of the midwife at work forms an informal aspect of the job description, and substantially defines the professional relationship between midwife and obstetrician (Willis, 1989). The professional subordination of midwives in Australia is especially pertinent given recent changes to legislation which brought midwives under the control of the Nurses Act. Although the NHMRC proposed a national register of midwives, midwives in Victoria, for example, are no longer recognized under the Act as specialist professionals, and may be seconded to any other area of hospital work.

The NHMRC Panel in the recent Australian report on options for the future did not address the question of direct-entry midwifery (whereby midwives are not required to obtain nursing qualifications prior to studying midwifery). This was a serious omission because direct-entry training effectively avoids the indoctrination of students into the medical model. The absence of direct-entry schemes and continued obstetric control over midwifery training and standards has meant that midwives have gradually lost their sense of professional autonomy and competence. This has been compounded by fragmented work practices in hospitals where midwives are divided into one of three areas: antenatal care, delivery or postnatal care. This lack of continuity has diluted their confidence to care for women in all phases of maternity without obstetric supervision and without resorting to high-technology monitoring and surveillance.

Maternal satisfaction

The NHRC report detailed what women wanted from a good birth: safety, control over the birth process, access to and sharing of information, and continuity of care. These were the conditions for positive birthing cited in the qualitative study of 40 women already mentioned, who gave birth at home or in hospital in Britain and Australia. However, the NHMRC report also noted that three state-based reports on maternity services in New South Wales, Victoria and Western Australia had concluded with the maxim that '...the majority were satisfied with the present provision of maternity services' (NHMRC, 1994). Significant qualification needs to be made on the basis of what the report understands as 'satisfactory' from the point of view of women. In the case of Victoria, the maternity satisfaction survey included only 1% of the birthing population. One could argue that this is not a representative sample, despite assertions to the contrary by the authors of the report.

The term 'satisfaction' is also open to question. For example, most of the 20 women in the qualitative study who gave birth in hospital reported that they were generally satisfied with the care they received. However, these women also reported that they did not *enjoy* their births. Most had desired no intervention and most received it. Typically, women who have given birth in hospital say that their ideal birth is a 'natural' birth, meaning little or no intervention, bar 'gas and air' if necessary. (I am using their terminology. Theoretically, it is understood that there is no such thing as a 'natural' birth, since all events are socially and culturally mediated. For example, a whisper of encouragement at the right time should be seen as a profound intervention.) On the other hand, the women said they would accept intervention if they were assured that it was absolutely necessary to ensure the safety of their baby. However, they invariably reported that under ideal conditions they would want to manage the birth themselves. By contrast, macrostatistical analysis shows that only a few will escape some chemical or surgical technique during their labour. Indeed, the Birthing Services Review (Department of Health, Victoria, 1990) showed that, of a sample of 100 women delivering in hospitals in Victoria, only 11% received no intervention.

Home birth in Australia

An expanded set of choices for women in Australia would also have included home birth, as it did in the Winterton Report in Britain. The Australian report was at best ambivalent and ultimately dismissive of this option. Although federal funding has been made available for pilot hombirth schemes in the USA, the NHMRC paper noted that home births in Australia (Bastian and Lancaster, 1992) had documented higher numbers of fetal deaths during labour compared to hospital births. A fuller account of these figures was subsequently furnished by Bastian and discussed by Bundy (1993). The figures show that deaths during labour accounted for 0.9 per 1000 births for national hospital rates as opposed to 2.4 per 1000 for home births. Overall, perinatal deaths (stillbirths plus neonatal deaths) were 4.8 per 1000 for home births compared with 3.7 per 1000 for national hospital rates. Apart from one birth (which was a preterm breech birth), the deaths at home (both antepartum and intrapartum) were due largely to asphyxia (lack of oxygen) or fetal distress in labour.

In response to the relative increase in intrapartum deaths at home, the NHMRC report effectively ruled out home birth on the grounds that it would require more than 700 000 women to be able to include 176 000 in a randomized trial to accurately assess the comparative mortality rates for home versus hospital delivery. No discussion was provided on the American, British and Dutch studies, which have argued that home birth is as safe as, or safer than, hospital birth (Tew, 1990; Tew and Damstra-Wijmenga, 1991; Durand, 1992; Campbell and Macfarlane, 1987). The NHMRC report acknowledged the credible work of Campbell and Macfarlane from the Oxford Epidemiology Unit in Britain, but did not say that the Campbell and Macfarlane study argued that there was no evidence that hospital delivery was safer than home birth. The NHMRC draft document failed to acknowledge the studies undertaken by Tew, whose work had incorporated extensive survey findings of comparative location carried out in Britain and in Holland (where over 30% of women continue to deliver at home). Tew concluded that infant mortality was lower at home at all levels of obstetric-defined risk, including the highest-risk categories. The dismissal of Tew's work may be traced to her central argument that frequent obstetric interventions have not reduced mortalities for which they have been imposed (Tew, 1990).

The report may have noted, as Bundy has done, that the excess of intra-partum deaths in Australia may have been avoided by a policy of continuous monitoring by a Pinard's fetal stethoscope or Sonicaid portable electronic monitoring device, and by early transfer to hospital where fetal distress was noted. The draft document might also have advocated direct-entry midwifery schemes where midwives would be trained as professionals in their own right, and the introduction of a policy which did not confer registration on midwives unless an agreed upon minimum number of births were attended per year. The report also failed to note that although home birth is not free from complications, the number of injuries recorded at home in one study were far less than those recorded by Mehl *et al.* in hospital deliveries (Bundy, 1993). The draft report might also have noted two studies of home birth carried out in Western Australia and in South Australia (Woodcock *et al.*, 1990). Although the SA study showed a PNMR adjusted for birthweight and lethal congenital abnormalities to be five times higher than among hospital births, close examination of the individual deaths concluded that the majority could not be directly attributed to the place of birth. The WA study reported a standardized rate of 4.03 per 1000 compared with an observed proportion of 5.05 per 1000. These rates are relatively favourable, especially when it is realized that not all the women were categorized as low-risk. Similarly, national PNMR rates which recorded more deaths at home had been standardized only for birthweight and congenital abnormalities, but not for maternal risk. It should be noted that Tew did calculate her results from fully standardized figures to show the greater safety of home birth over hospital birth at every level of maternal risk.

The conclusion to be drawn from these studies is that:

- proper training and accreditation procedures be required of independent midwives;
- that appropriate transfer policies be set in place;
- that adequate medical back-up be made available in the community to assist home births;
- that appropriate selection criteria be placed upon women intending to give birth at home;
- that women intending to give birth at home must be prepared to accept due responsibility for an unexpected outcome.

Finally, it must be pointed out that in a very few cases, even when the above criteria are observed, mortality cannot be avoided, whether in hospital or at home. It is interesting for a researcher to observe that until very recently, the high rates of intervention and morbidity associated with hospital births have rarely been questioned. Yet the relatively low rates of home-birth mortality have been subjected to major inquisition.

BIRTH AS EUPHORIA

When 20 women in Britain and Australia were asked what they liked about home birth they nominated control over procedures and conditions, continuity of care, peaceful and familiar environment, family support and security of the birthplace. These were the conditions for positive birthing and they were mentioned in both British and Australian policy documents as being important for all women, regardless of location of delivery. Most of the 20 women who gave birth in hospital in either Britain or Australia also cited such conditions as being germane to positive birthing, whether or not they experienced the conditions during their birth.

Why then bother with pursuing the question of home birth when a birthing centre, like Moorabin (described above), adopting a non-interventionist and client-centred model of care, could very nearly equate with the desires and expectations of most women? In other words, if you just asked women what were the conditions for positive birthing it is immanently possible to achieve them in a birthing centre adopting a client-centred philosophy.

However, it is argued here that home birth offers a qualitatively different experience for women: it is euphoric. Further, unlike the women who had hospital births, some home-birthing women tend to report a significant shift in self-identity as a result of their birthing experience. For example, the following comments were made about the birth experience:

> I cried and cried, because it was just so wonderful. We all did. And I felt, I think felt stronger after that in myself, my own character, because I achieved this on my own. [I felt stronger in] relationships with other people and [now] I feel free to talk to people. I have an inner strength and that comes across in all areas, relationships, within family, and with outside people. A strength within myself that I know that I can do anything now, or not anything, but the confidence. I can go out and I can achieve that. I have a strength that I never had before, because to have a birth at home in my own bedroom, that was a strength. (Meredith)
>
> It [the homebirth] was the most transforming thing that has ever happened to me. I have changed incredibly since the birth of my

children especially now [since the homebirth]. I was brought up I think to respect authority...I suppose you could put me under being 'radical' now, compared to other women...We [who birthed at home] don't tend to tell our birthing stories to many women because it's often met with I think a little bit of hostility because they say how bad their labour was – the pain was unbearable, the forceps delivery and everything. I think we've had such wonderful births. It was fantastic. Other women tend to dislike the minority group.

[The major difference between the first hospital birth and the second homebirth] would have been just being so at ease and I think I was in my premium environment really where I didn't have to worry about anyone else. I didn't have to worry about people's, you know, that midwife I just remember that look on her face and things like that. I was totally absorbed in myself being at home. There were no distractions. I could totally concentrate by myself. (Susan)

I was just on top of it. It was more a mental thing. I could cope with it. I have never really thought about it. It was wonderful. Everything went well. I couldn't have asked for a better birth. And I guess I compared it to Kylie's birth [in hospital] and thought this is better than anything. [Anne thought her hospital birth had been 'fine']. The feeling – I felt different too after that [the homebirth]...it gave me a lot more strength. It made me feel really good. Not just about my body. About me, that I could do this. I was more than an achievement. I can't explain it. It's an inner thing. I think I am a lot stronger after it. (Anne)

It is a spiritual process, an emotional process. It's putting me and the baby in our place within humanity if you like. It might sound a bit crazy, but I feel that when I give birth I am doing something that women did thousands and thousands of years ago...birth is one thing we still have in common with our ancestors going back to the beginning of time. I think probably giving birth to the children, is very important. It goes to the very top of the list of my achievements if you like. (Dianne)

If I did it again I would make sure that I got the dim lights and the quietness...For me the best part of the home birth was the continuity of care and being in my own home in my own territory. I mean what better place to be born, everybody should have their right to be born in the place where they belong. In the final analysis I felt that best part about home birth was when everybody had gone home and we just crawled into bed. The three of us just laid in bed together and thought how clever we were. What wonderful people we were. (Renate)

[Caroline considered that she had had 'a wonderful birth' in a birthing centre for her second baby. She had experienced continuity of care with a known midwife, she was the only woman in the unit, there was freedom of mobility and choice of delivery position. She described that birth as 'a totally empowering feeling'. She described that second birth in hospital as 'the most satisfying']:

> I had a much stronger sense of sisterhood and being a woman and I felt like a woman and I think I just had that really strong sense if you can't be a woman when you are giving birth, and so on, whenever can you be. I'd had the opportunity and set up a situation where I was able to do that and yet I feel that is taken away from so many women and they are made to feel like little girls, when they are in this vulnerable yet wonderfully empowering position.

Of the home birth, in comparison, she said:

> It was like the icing on the cake because it was where it should be and it was great. (Caroline)
>
> Well, prior to Jenny's birth I felt like a non-person. I really didn't feel like anything. I sort of had a lot of problems with my identity as such. It wasn't really until Jenny's birth that I thought, yes, I am a woman. This is what women are supposed to do. This is really great. Whereas prior to that, I wasn't really sure. I just was really lost and I'm sure it was because I hadn't had a very good experience as a woman, as being a woman in a woman's body should have, I guess. (Jessica)
>
> It was good, it was just all round everything, it was a natural birth, it was the way that your body had meant it to be. There was no intervention and I think it was just so reassuring for [the midwife] to empower me to say you know what you want, you know what your body wants, go with your body. (Isabella)
>
> I mean if you have a baby and you can say that you've done that well, it's going to reflect on whatever else you are going to do after that because you have already got that high self-esteem and self-achievement and you can move on to something else and know that you can do that just as well. I am not saying that everyone has to have a baby at home in order to achieve that. You can have high self-achievement in hospital as well, as long as you can keep the professional people who are willing to hear what you want and not what they're willing to do to you. (Tania)
>
> Looking after women as a midwife I felt that a lot of women lost control and they lost their dignity as well [in hospital], which really upset me. ....especially with public patients right from the word go from the first time they go to the antenatal clinic, they are just sort of treated as a piece of meat almost. They [the doctors] look at the uterus and the birth canal and that's it. .. they don't look at the

woman. Also, if it was the natural, normal sort of life event why go into hospital. Hospital is for sick people, that's how I saw it.

My whole body was sort of warm with love and it was really nice and being at home and being in my own environment was just nice and it was so quiet. I felt the birth was just an amazing achievement for me. It was just the ultimate achievement for my self-confidence, I think. I felt so confident afterwards...it just boosted me. I just felt wonderful, I felt confident, I felt I could just about face anything. And things that used to bother me after the birth of my first child [at home]...well, if this person doesn't like me for whatever reason, it's their bad luck. I'm a wonderful person, whereas before it would worry me. (Deborah)

[The home birth was] extremely good. I am a very strong believer that that positive launch into motherhood, into parenthood, into the world for the baby, is like the crest of a wave that helps to carry you along for quite a long time. And I think if you don't have that, for those who've had difficult and traumatic births, I think they're struggling. They haven't got that crest of a wave, and they're struggling for a long time afterwards, sometimes forever. It colours their whole attitude towards their child or children, parenthood. And I think that I had that crest of a wave [after the home birth]. Okay, I had ups and downs afterwards, but I really feel that on the crest of the wave I was launched. (Janet)

CONCLUSION

It has been argued that Australian birthing policies are retrogressive compared to recent policy changes in Britain. First, home birth received scant attention from the Australian NHMRC (1994), ostensibly on the grounds that it cannot be assessed accurately by prospective randomized controlled trials. Retrospective trials in Australia have pointed to fairly good outcomes compared with semistandardized comparisons with hospital births on national and state scales. Several large overseas studies support the view that home birth may be safer: conservative findings report that it is at least as safe as hospital birth. Although intrapartum care and training procedures for Australian midwives might receive more attention in policy recommendations, the ultimate censoring of home birth is not warranted. First, women will continue to give birth at home. These women will continue to be disadvantaged unless policies are put into place to ensure adequate back-up in the community and to ensure rapid transfer to hospital in emergency cases. In addition, the censoring of home birth does not fulfil the NHMRC's stated aim of increasing the range of options and models of care for Australian women.

Second, quantitative methodologies related to women's experiences of birthing at home and in hospital cannot fully comprehend the complexities and contradictions in the phenomenological aspects of the birthing experience. Women who give birth in hospital may report a 'satisfactory' rating on a standardized questionnaire, but when questioned in depth about their experience, most will report serious anomalies with the event as a whole. The NHMRC's assumption that most women viewed existing hospital practices as satisfactory does not stand up to qualitative inquiry. Further, sole reliance on evidence gleaned from randomized control trials on the grounds that this methodology will be certain to yield an unbiased scientific truth cannot be supported. When used to assess interventions, the method is unethical (how does one exclude someone who is in need of a caesarean?), and nor is the method comprehensive. For example, it is designed to test only one variable. Birthing is a complex set of interrelated events which cannot be discretely separated and measured. The events are also cumulative – positively or negatively. In the latter case, the 'cascade of intervention' is a prime example (Department of Health, Victoria, 1990; World Health Organization, 1985). Further, in the case of randomized controlled trials, the variable which is screened out for measurement may well be the primary causal factor, which itself should be assessed in its interrelation with other factors. In the case of phenomenological factors discussed above, this criticism must certainly hold. As Richards (1991) has argued, there are no 'objective' measures, whether posited from randomized controlled trials or qualitative studies, and no methodology can expunge evaluator bias either in the design of the project or its assessement. There are only stories, patterns and trends. The findings from qualitative studies reported in this paper point to the idiosyncratic nature of the birthing process, precisely because women interpret their social and physical environment in diverse and unpredictable ways. Any democratic and humane maternity system must accommodate a great degree of idiosyncracy as the one 'certainty'. That is, although women in the present study reported the four conditions for positive birthing – continuity of care, control over procedures and conditions, and safety and peace in the birthplace – exactly how these were translated into specific measures remained open to individual interpretation. For example, some women wanted to be able to move around, some wanted to get into the bath, some wanted back rubs, some wanted to be left alone with their partner but with the midwife close by, and others wanted the midwife to be with them all of the time.

Third, the women who gave birth at home reported substantially different experiences. It is not an overstatement to describe their evaluations as euphoric. Such women reported that birthing represented for them an act of universal human creativity, an opportunity for positive transformation in self-identity, and an apogee in the rites of passage of the human lifecycle. They did not assess birthing in those terms when the location had been hospital and when the care they received included routine interventions under an orthodox obstetric philosophy.

Fourth, and finally, it is a politically defined assumption to posit birthing as a choice between safety (hospital) and ecstasy (home). A social model of birthing sees affective states as a critical precondition for ease of birthing and positive outcome for both mother and child. The positive conditions of birthing are best met either at home or in an independent birthing centre, staffed entirely by midwives and employing a woman-centred philosophy which guarantees control by women over conditions and procedures, peace and security and continuity of care.

Although the NHMRC recommendations appeared to negate an orthodox medical model, it is predicted that obstetric dominance will not subside in the short or longer term. Women will continue to opt for obstetric care in hospital because medical power has successfully instituted a view of birthing as a hazardous and dangerous process. Thus, to a certain extent, Beck (1992) has been correct to argue that medicine is an extreme case of sub-politics. Beck argued that although other areas of science are increasingly open to public criticism, successful professionalization of medicine since the turn of the century has prevented its delegitimation, both internally and externally. This is because medicine has been able to protect its research institutionally, it has been able to determine its own standards and training procedures for future generations of students, and it has been able to control the practical application of the knowledge within its own institutions – the clinics. The medical profession has been able to convince the public that it is conceptually uninformed and that it lags hopelessly behind medical innovation and medical knowledge. Finally, Beck argued, control over nature has in consequence achieved complete mastery over the subject.

Both Beck (1992) and Foucault (1973) agree that medicine is a parable about social control. This paper supports that conclusion. Yet Beck's analysis of the impenetrable nature of medical science cannot be entirely supported. Significant changes have occurred in birthing practices and current policy initiatives have challenged obstetric dominance, especially in Britain. I have described the British system as a bifurcated model because recent policy initiatives have posed a serious challenge to orthodox systems, but I do not wish to be overly optimistic here. The medical model remains dominant despite the challenges. In other words, there is still a gap between discourses about woman-centred alternative models and the practice. For example, there is no guarantee that midwife-run practices will adopt a social model. Nor is it a certainty that women will attend such practices in the same numbers as those seeking conventional obstetric care in hospitals. At the most, we would expect a gradual move towards midwife-only care and probably more so among white, Anglo-Saxon and more highly educated women (Bastian, 1992). Disadvantaged and minority groups who are not so aware of alternatives will continue to attend hospitals and receive orthodox care, and experience high levels of intervention typical of that model of care. Further, the medical model has consolidated its dominance within childbirth in Britain over the past 40 years. It may take at least this time to construct and consolidate an alternative, if not longer.

The Australian case is even less positive than the British situation. Although the recent policy document published by the NHMRC purported to be critical of medical models of birthing, the new arrangements will fall far short of any real challenge to existing forms of social control.

AUTHOR'S NOTE

This research was funded by a Deakin University Research Development Fellowship granted in 1993. I am indebted to my mentor, Professor Robyn Rowland, for her academic support, collegiality and friendship in making this project possible.

REFERENCES

Bastian, H. (1992) *Who Gives Birth at Home and Why?*, Canberra, Homebirth Australia Inc.

Bastian, H. and Lancaster, P.A.L. (1992) *Home Births in Australia 1988–1990*, AIHW National Perinatal Statistics Unit, Sydney.

Beck, U. (1992) *Risk Society: Towards a New Modernity*, Sage Publications, London.

Biro, M.-A. and Lumley, J. (1991) The safety of team midwifery: the first decade of the Monash Birth Centre. *Medical Journal of Australia* 155, 478–80.

Bundy, J. (1993) *Home Birth – Why Not?: Observations of an Obstetrician*, Published by the author, Australia.

Campbell, R. and Macfarlane, A. (1987) *Where to be Born: the Debate and the Evidence*, National Perinatal Epidemiology Unit, Oxford.

Chalmers, I. (1978) Implications of the current debate on obstetric practice, in *The Place of Birth*, ed S. Kitzinger, Oxford University Press, Oxford, pp.44–54.

Crotty, M., Ramsay, A.T., Smart, R. and Chan, A. (1990) Planned homebirths in South Australia 1976–1987. *Medical Journal of Australia* 153, 664–7.

Douglas, M. (1990) Risk as a forensic resource. *Daedalus*, Fall, 1–16.

Durand, A.M. (1992) The safety of home birth: the farm study. *American Journal of Public Health* 82(3), 450–3.

Elliott, C.E. (1992) Obstetrics in a small maternity hospital. *Australian Family Physician*, May 21,(5), 613–9.

Foucault, M. (1973) *The Birth of the Clinic*, Tavistock, London.

Winterton Committee (House of Commons, Great Britain) (1992) *Maternity Services: Second Report*, Vol. 1, HMSO, London.

Department of Health, Victoria (1990) *Final Report of the Ministerial Review of Birthing Services in Victoria: Having a Baby in Victoria*, Department of Health, Victoria.

Klein, M., Lloyd, I., Redman, C. *et al.* (1983) A comparison of low-risk pregnant women booked for delivery in two systems of care: shared care (consultant) and integrated general practice unit. I Obstetric procedures and newborn outcomes, and II Labour and delivery management and neonatal outcome. *British Journal of Obstetrics and Gynaecology* **90**, 118–20 and 123–8.

Linder-Pelz, S., Webster, M.A., Martins, J. and Greenwell, J. (1990) Obstetric risks and outcomes: birth centre compared with conventional labour ward. *Community Health Studies* **XIV**(1), 39–46.

Marsden, W. (1994) *Pursuing the Birth Machine: the Search for Appropriate Birth Technology*, ACE Graphics, Australia.

Morris, N., Campbell, J., Biro, M-A. *et al.* (1986) Birth centre confinement at the Queen Victoria Medical Centre: four years' experience. *Medical Journal of Australia* **144**, 628–30.

National Health and Medical Research Council of Australia, Health Care Committee (1994) *Options for Effective Care in Childbirth: Consultation Document*, NHMRC, Canberra.

Oakley, A. (1986) *The Captured Womb: a History of the Medical Care of Pregnant Women*, Basil Blackwell, Oxford.

Permezel, J.M.H., Pepperel, R.J. and Kloss, M. (1987) Unexpected problems in patients selected for birthing unit delivery. *Australian and New Zealand Journal of Obstetrics and Gynaecology* **27**, 21–3.

Richards, E. (1991) *Vitamin C and Cancer: Medicine or Politics?*, Macmillan, Australia.

Tew, M. (1990) *Safer Childbirth? A Critical History of Maternity Care*, Chapman & Hall, London.

Tew, M. and Damstra-Wijmenga, S.M.I. (1991) Safest birth attendants: recent Dutch evidence. *Midwifery* **7**, 55–63.

Turner, B.S. (1987) *Medical Power and Social Knowledge*, Sage Publications, London.

Willis, E. (1989) *Medical Dominance: the Division of Labour in Australian Health Care*, Allen and Unwin, Sydney.

Woodcock, H.C., Read, A.W., Moore, D.J. *et al.*(1990) Planned homebirths in Western Australia 1981–1987: a descriptive study. *Medical Journal of Australia* **153**, 672–8.

World Health Organization (1985) *Having a Baby in Europe: Report on a Study, Public Health in Europe 26*, World Health Organization, Copenhagen.

CHAPTER 11

Intervention or understanding: the uses of applied nutrition research

Pat Crotty

INTRODUCTION

Dietary reform is widely assumed to be the justification for investigating food behaviour and dietary intake. As a consequence nutrition education is usually deemed unsuccessful when dietary change is not achieved. An excessively narrow orientation to dietary reform in both nutrition theory and practice limits the possibilities for developing research which illuminates food behaviour and consumption for its own sake.

The disciplines of social nutrition and nutritional anthropology, although they may produce data useful in interventions, should not be constrained by contemporary normative ideas of 'good' nutrition. This paper examines these disciplines and discusses the breadth of questions they address, some of the methodologies which are currently in use and the insights being generated through their application.

In 1981 Paul Rozin published an amusing and insightful allegory for nutrition's 'two cultures', in which extraterrestrials from the 'Martian Institute' or 'Foundation for Furthering Science' (MIFFS, Earth Sport Section) discuss how they might conduct research to understand the human phenomenon of football (gridiron), having concentrated their research efforts on tennis for the past decade. Those scientists who have developed quite some expertise in researching tennis are upset that funds might be diverted from their area, particularly since there are a number of interesting issues still unresolved, for example they know that yellow balls are used sometimes but are unable to predict their use. Pigment analysis studies have only just started.

In allocating funds to the new studies a MIFFS research committee must decide between a number of different approaches: for example, one observation is that the six humans dressed in black and white stripes who are on the field at all times represent the essential element of the game. Others on the committee believe that the 'ellipsoidal object' sometimes observed in the game is its focus; others disagree on the basis that the object is not seen very much and therefore probably does not matter. The committee hears another view that players grouping closely together seemed to be the essential element of the game, as subsequently there is random activity where players run in different directions and seem to 'let off steam'. Studying player grouping was eventually agreed to be the approach most likely to be successful. Suggested methodological approaches to these studies included, using quantifiable aspects of the game, for example players' numbers plotted against their position in the close group configuration.

In making its funding decision one research approach was rejected because it was not based on objective and quantifiable data collection; the researchers concerned proposed merely to observe the general flow of the game:

> '...and to supplement and guide these observations with interviews of the players, in an attempt to find out what the game was about. They proposed to ask players such open-ended questions as: What is the purpose of this game? Is the ball important? and Why do the players move to one end of the field and then to the other? (Rozin, 1981)

The committee questioned the reliability of the data in particular verbal reports:

> Why for example, should one believe a player's claim that he moved to the right to misdirect other players or that the rarely visible ball was the centre of activity? (Rozin, 1981)

Through this allegory Rozin draws a picture of our understanding of food selection as being at the early stage of 'understanding the game'. Food selection and the influences on it, he suggests, are so poorly understood that much of the work that is currently needed must be conducted within the traditions of the social sciences. Rozin goes on to discuss the nature of research problems and methods appropriate to the study of food selection. He supports the conduct of descriptive studies and warns against premature quantification, pointing out that progress cannot be assumed just because something can be counted.

The focus of what follows is on the disciplines and methodologies which have made some inroads into the study of human food selection and consumption at the level of 'understanding the game'. It is possible to argue that nutrition should leave such work to social scientists and concentrate at the level of foods, the nutrients they contain and the consequences of their consumption. Elsewhere I have characterized this direction as 'post-swallowing nutrition' (as distinct from 'pre-swallowing nutrition'), and argued that although they may occupy different paradigmatic spaces, it is essential there is a bridge between the two which must remain in good order if public health nutrition policies and nutrition education programmes are to be morally defensible (Crotty, 1992, 1995).

COMBINING THE NATURAL AND SOCIAL SCIENCES IN NUTRITION RESEARCH

The two best-known disciplines which connect the social and natural sciences in nutrition are social nutrition and nutritional anthropology. Social nutrition is associated with the United Kingdom and nutritional anthropology, particularly its more cultural version, is North American in origin. A more biologically orientated version of nutritional anthropology is associated with Cambridge University (Ulijaszek and Strickland, 1993).

McKenzie (1980) defined social nutrition as '...the study of the social, psychological and economic factors that determine food habits, and of the means by which future choice may be influenced in the interests of better nutrition'.

Nutritional anthropology has been described as 'an umbrella term which includes sociocultural, biocultural and physical (or biological) anthropology' (Weinstein, 1980) and its outcomes as 'a body of data and theory on the relationships of nutrition to sociocultural, economic, and ecological processes' (Pelto, 1989).

In a recent text on research methods within the discipline, the practical applications of nutritional anthropology are clearly demonstrated (Pelto *et al.*, 1989). One of the important influences on the development of the field has been its practical focus. This has produced a tension between the traditional anthropological approaches of fieldwork, which may last a year or more, and the needs of policy makers and workers in the field who may require essential background information in a particular setting to ensure the practicality and success of interventions. By and large nutritional anthropology has made contributions in such situations by ensuring the collection of specific dietary data against a background of general ethnographic information, using both qualitative and quantitative methods. This has made an impact on methods used in nutrition surveys and in nutritional epidemiology, and has been useful in community nutrition studies and nutrition planning.

More recently, Sobal (1992) has defined a new subdiscipline, nutritional sociology, as '...the application of sociological theories and methods to examining and influencing food patterns, eating habits, and nutrition'. Both McKenzie's and Sobal's definitions give prominence to social nutrition's and nutritional sociology's roles in interventions in dietary change efforts. Nutritional anthropology also has an increasingly well documented track record of practicality in the field.

Sociological Approaches

From a sociological perspective, Mennel *et al.* (1992), in reviewing the growing literature studying eating, diet and culture, note the diversity both of theoretical perspectives from which food selection has been studied and the issues which have become the focus for sociocultural approaches. The development of culinary cultures; lay perspectives on food and health; the impact of colonialism and migration on food patterns; domestic food preparation and distribution; and the influences of industrialization and food technology on food supplies are some of the issues discussed. They also note the related research networks established around particular groups. Among these networks they nominate Paris as being particularly well endowed with outstanding researchers, including Claude Fischler (Fischler, 1993) and the Food and Society group in the United States which includes Whit and McIntosh (Sobal *et al.*, 1993).

Australia has yet to develop a strong research focus in the sociocultural aspects of food and nutrition, although there have been some notable related contributions. There is in Australia a lively interest in gastronomy and multiculturalism in food (Symons, 1993) and some major biomedical nutrition studies which have integrated cultural background with research into food and nutrient consumption (Powles *et al.*, 1988; Lee *et al.*, 1994; O'Dea, 1994). However, from within the research tradition of nutrition the most frequent focus of studies is still rather narrowly that of food as a source of nutrients and the biomedical consequences of consumption. The most likely explanation for this focus is the underlying intention to eventually, if not immediately, apply the knowledge in health promoting interventions which assume dietary reform. However, as Cassidy (1994) has pointed out, even if a study is sited very specifically within the biomedical paradigm, recognition of the importance of sociocultural factors may make the difference between useful interpretations of dietary data and potentially damaging ones.

Whatever variations there may be within these disciplines, for example whether they adopt a structuralist or a materialist ideology, or whether they direct their efforts towards the practice of anthropology or sociology in nutrition or towards the development of the anthropology or sociology of food and nutrition (Sobal, 1992), their theoretical perspectives emphasize the link between food behaviour and practices and their social context (Murcott, 1988).

NUTRITIONAL ANTHROPOLOGY

Studies of Dietary Intake

The gathering of information about food consumed is a central task for nutrition, whether a study is biomedically defined or is more orientated towards sociocultural concerns. Cassidy (1994) has recently noted that, traditionally, nutritionists and epidemiologists have not been very concerned with aspects of meaning such as world views or explanatory models, despite the fact that the meanings that people ascribe to food and food behaviour may have consequences for the collection of dietary data. A well validated and reliable questionnaire conforming to the requirements of scientific method, may nevertheless exacerbate problems of cultural distance between researcher and respondent. Cassidy (1994) gives the example of cross-cultural work, where meanings given to the word 'food' may vary between researchers and their respondents. In some cultures '...people distinguish 'food' from 'sauce': food is the grain staple and sauce is everything else. A false view of diet as tremendously limited could emerge if researchers asked people to report their food intake without also asking about their sauce intake'.

Many such problems can be overcome or at least reduced by careful listening, for example in small groups such as focus group discussions, and by taking in as much information about local food use as possible. This could include participation in local food activities such as shopping and festivities, as well as interviewing informants. The information gathered in these ways can be used in constructing more formal questionnaires or surveys. However, in an interesting reversal of the usual relationship between qualitative and quantitative data in nutrition research, Cassidy asserts the primacy of the qualitative data in validating the quantitative:

> ...the accuracy of the quantitative step is proven when and if the quantitative data gathered from a large sample closely resemble the qualitative data gathered in the same population from a small sample. This point is emphasized because many researchers incorrectly assume that quantitative data are more accurate than qualitative data, or that quantifiable data are explanatory, when, in fact they are descriptive. (Cassidy, 1994)

In another argument the idea of a 'gold standard' dietary assessment method which produces valid and reliable data in a range of circumstances is questioned. Cassidy's argument is that ultimately, if a study is making comparisons across cultures, what will be compared is the outcome of the dietary assessment, and the important problem to solve is that the particular method (e.g. 24-hour recall) works well, that is, it yields good-quality information for the particular situation under study. This then allows for adjusting the format of the method to fit particular circumstances, e.g. a 24-hour recall could be administered by computer, in written form or by interview.

In addition to integrating sociocultural concerns into traditional nutrition research methodologies, nutritional anthropology in particular has contributed important new concepts and approaches to the study of food and nutrition. These approaches belong in the category of both studies of food and nutrition and studies within nutrition. Growing interest in the processes surrounding nutrition, such as dietary change, may further promote them (Rotberg and Rabb, 1985).

Freedom from some of the epistemological constraints of studies within biological nutrition facilitates a shift in focus from individuals to social units, such as households, from nutrients and foods to meals and menus, and from biochemistry of bodies to the relationships which surround eating and the activities of everyday life on which feeding and eating depend. The phenomena which become a focus for sociocultural approaches and the research methodologies appropriate to their study are just as important as the biomedical considerations – in fact, in terms of problem definition and programme planning they may be much more so.

For example, Goode (1989) has identified extrinsic and intrinsic factors which affect both individual and group food choices through what she calls 'culinary behaviours'. These include food availability (which is itself a product of prior factors, such as how food is produced and distributed); accessibility of food, which involves the effort necessary to get to and from a food supply and the cost of the food itself; the various aspects of provisioning, such as food storage, cooking fuel, equipment and facilities; and the more cultural influences, such as ideas of etiquette and behaviour during eating and the structuring of meals themselves.

Rapid Assessment Procedures (RAPs)

One of the most interesting recent developments in the methodological area has been the application of rapid assessment procedures to nutrition. This is currently focused almost exclusively on developing countries, but its broader application in industrialized countries has the potential to radically alter what is currently thought of as community or public health nutrition. It could offer a coherent set of methods and strategies which integrates qualitative and quantitative methodologies and an underlying philosophy consistent with cultural sensitivity in both research and practice. This is currently a great need in developed countries, given the contemporary emphasis on biomedically driven, universally applied dietary reform, particularly through the international promulgation of culturally homogenous dietary guidelines. RAPs may offer a package which can encompass and apply in appropriate circumstances all those factors influencing food selection, as well as the methodological approaches which have been included here under the sociocultural category.

These techniques of data gathering and interpretation have developed particularly in the past decade, and address circumstances where little time or other resources are available. In their original form of rapid rural appraisal they were necessitated by a serious shortage of social knowledge in development interventions (Cernea, 1992). They may now include a wide range of innovative strategies, such as group interviews, mapping, role playing and forms of participant observation as well as the use of secondary sources of information. Various forms of traditional dietary data collection can be incorporated when used for food and nutrition-related problems. Scrimshaw (1992) notes the essential characteristics of this approach as:

- striving to be rapid and practical for problem solving;
- using a number of sources of information in providing accurate data;
- paying less heed than usual to the boundaries between research, practice, community participation and community development.

Very practical guidelines for the implementation of this approach have been available for some time and cover everything from how to deal with field notes, map social relationships, run focus groups and collect and analyse data (Scrimshaw and Hurtado, 1987).

Health workers who conduct community-wide cardiovascular disease risk factor reduction programmes at the local level have recently been encouraged to adopt a year-long community assessment process, so crucial does community organization seem to be for the success of such programmes (Mittelmark *et al.*,1993). Rapid assessment procedures would seem to be eminently adaptable to such circumstances.

A CASE IN POINT

Most of the developmental thinking about socially sensitive food habit research methods and attempts to understand the nature of food selection are embedded in a background of development problems from the third world. It may be easier to see sociocultural issues in nutrition as an 'outsider': perhaps this is why there are notable unexplored examples in our own society, where these methods are eminently applicable and yet very traditional socially insensitive nutrition research methods are applied.

The food choices of low-income Australians have frequently been identified as problematic, never more so since the conflation of the inequitous distribution of coronary disease mortality with unsubstantiated views about the capacity of poor families to choose food 'wisely'. An important part of the contemporary explanation of higher rates of heart disease among the less affluent is said to be their choice of a less healthy diet than the more affluent. An unhappy mixture of fact and prejudice about poverty and poor people, combined with the assumption that 'healthy eating' as currently defined is an unmitigated good, has masked the very real possibility that healthy eating is more expensive than most people's current food choices. For example, direct substitution of higher-fat products by the reduced-fat varieties can indeed increase food costs (Wilson, 1989; Cade and Booth, 1990; Maggiore, 1991; McAllister *et al.*, 1994). One reading of McAllister *et al.*'s study is that if low-income families wish to follow current guidelines (which very few people in any income category currently achieve) without incurring greater food expenses, they may have to make major changes to their dietary choices, in particular to curtail what may be considered as spending on 'recreational' foods such as cakes and biscuits. This area would seem to be wide open to applying the kinds of research strategies discussed above. First, trying to understand from the insider's perspective what it is like to feed a family on a small amount of money. The use of these research strategies can develop respect for the accommodations people make to their social environment, even if it contradicts the experts' wisdom. For example, while it is widely advocated that a way of saving money is to buy foods on special offer, women respond in different ways to special offers, from enthusiastically pursuing them to weighing up whether it is worth the time, effort and transport costs to seek them out.

CONCLUSION

The proposal of the title represents an unsatisfactory dichotomy. The study of 'meaning' and 'values' in nutrition is equally important to good qualitative and quantitative research in applied nutrition, whether it is for 'understanding the game' or for the planning and evaluation of nutrition interventions (Mittelmark *et al.*, 1993). In addition, there are aspects of current public health nutrition policies and programmes, from their unrecognized ethical dimensions (Skrabanek, 1990) to the need for new approaches to gathering information, which better serve initiatives in the new public health (Dean, 1994; Krieger, 1994; WHO, 1994). Researchers, practitioners and the wider community will all be better served by nutrition research approaches which place food selection in its widest possible social context.

REFERENCES

Cade, J. and Booth, S. (1990) What can people eat to meet the dietary goals: and how much does it cost? *Journal of Human Nutrition and Dietetics* 3, 199–207.
Cassidy, C.M. (1994) Walk a mile in my shoes: culturally sensitive food-habit research. *American Journal of Clinical Nutrition* 59(Suppl), 190S–7S.
Cernea, M.M. (1992) Re-tooling in applied social investigation for development planning: some methodological issues, in *Rapid Assessment Procedures: Qualitative Methodologies for Planning and Evaluation of Health Related Programmes*, eds N.S. Scrimshaw and G.R. Gleason, International Nutrition Foundation for Developing Countries, Boston, pp. 11–23.
Crotty, P. (1992) The value of qualitative research in nutrition. *Annual Review of Health Social Science* 3, 109–18.
Crotty, P. (1995) *Good Nutrition: Science or Culture?*, Allen and Unwin, Sydney.

Dean, K. (1994) Creating a new knowledge base for the new public health. *Journal of Epidemiology and Community Health* **48**, 217–19.

Fischler, C. (1993) A nutritional cacophony or the crisis of food selection in affluent societies, in *For a Better Nutrition in the 21st Century*, eds P. Leathwood, M. Horisberger and W.P.T. James, Raven Press, New York, pp. 57–65.

Goode, J. (1989) Cultural patterning and group-shared rules in the study of food intake, in *Research Methods in Nutritional Anthropology*, eds G.H. Pelto, P.J. Pelto and E. Messer, United Nations University, Tokyo, pp. 126–61.

Krieger, N. (1994) Epidemiology and the web of causation: has anyone seen the spider? *Social Science and Medicine* **39**(7), 887–903.

Lee, A.J., O'Dea, K. and Mathews, J.D. (1994) Apparent dietary intake in remote aboriginal communities. *Australian Journal of Public Health* **18**(2), 190–7.

Maggiore, P. (1991) Is a healthy diet affordable for families on a low income? *Australian Journal of Nutrition and Dietetics* **48**(2), 38–9.

McAllister, M., Baghurst, K. and Record, S. (1994) Financial costs of healthful eating: a comparison of three different approaches. *Journal of Nutrition Education* **26**, 131–9.

McKenzie, J. (1980) What is social nutrition? *BNF Nutrition Bulletin* **5**(6), 309–25.

Mennel, S., Murcott, A. and van Oterloo, A.H. (1992) *The Sociology of Food:Eating, Diet and Culture*, Sage Publications, London.

Mittelmark, M.B., Hunt, M.K., Heath, G.W. and Schmid, T.L. (1993) Realistic outcomes: lessons from community-based research and demonstration programmes for the prevention of cardiovascular diseases. *Journal of Public Health Policy* **144**, 437–62.

Murcott, A. (1988) Sociological and social anthropological approaches to food and eating, in *World Review of Nutrition and Dietetics, vol 55: Sociological and Medical Aspects of Nutrition*, ed G.H. Bourne, Karger, Basel, pp. 1–40.

O'Dea, K. (1994) The therapeutic and preventive potential of the hunter–gatherer lifestyle: insights from Australian Aborigines, in *Western Diseases: Their Dietary Prevention and Reversibility*, eds N.J. Temple and D.P. Burkitt, Humana, Totowa NJ, pp. 349–380.

Pelto, G.H. (1989) Introduction: methodological directions in nutritional anthropology, in *Research Methods in Nutritional Anthropology*, eds G.H. Pelto, P.J. Pelto and E. Messer, United Nations University, Tokyo, pp. ix–xvi.

Pelto, G.H., Pelto, P.J. and Messer, E. (eds) (1989) *Research Methods in Nutritional Anthropology*, United Nations University, Tokyo.

Powles, J., Ktenas, D., Sutherland, C. and Hage, B. (1988) Food habits in southern-European migrants: a case-study of migrants from the Greek island of Levkada, in *Food Habits in Australia. The First Deakin/Sydney Universities Symposium on Australian Nutrition*, eds A.S. Truswell and M.L. Wahlqvist, Rene Gordon, North Balwyn, pp. 201–23.

Rotberg, R. and Rabb, T.K. (eds) (1985) *Hunger and History: The Impact of Changing Food Production and Consumption Patterns on Society*, Cambridge University Press, Cambridge.

Rozin, P. (1981) The study of human food selection and the problems of 'Stage 1 Science', in *Nutrition and Behavior*, ed S.A. Miller, Franklin Institute Press, Philadelphia, pp. 9–18.

Scrimshaw, S.C.M. (1992) Adaptation of anthropological methodologies to rapid assessment of nutrition and primary health care, in *Rapid Assessment Procedures: Qualitative Methodologies for Planning and Evaluation of Health Related Programmes*, eds N.S. Scrimshaw and G.R. Gleason, International Nutrition Foundation for Developing Countries, Boston, pp. 25–38.

Scrimshaw, S.C.M. and Hurtado, E. (1987) *Rapid Assessment Procedures for Nutrition and Primary Health Care: Anthropological Approaches to Improving Programme Effectiveness*, United Nations University, Tokyo; UNICEF and the UCLA Latin American Center, Los Angeles.

Skrabanek, P. (1990) Why is preventive medicine exempted from ethical constraints? *Journal of Medical Ethics* **16**, 187–90.

Sobal, J. (1993) The practice of nutritional sociology. *Sociological Practice Review* **3**(1), 22–31.

Sobal, J., McIntosh, W.A. and Whit, W. (1992) Teaching the sociology of food, eating and nutrition. *Teaching Sociology* **21**(1), 50–9.

Symons, M. (1993) *The Shared Table*, AGPS, Canberra.

Ulijaszek, S.J. and Strickland, S.S. (1993) *Nutritional Anthropology: Prospects and Perspectives*, Smith-Gordon, London.

Weinstein, R.S. (1980) Defining nutritional anthropology. *Journal of Nutrition Education* **12**(4), 185–6.

Wilson, G. (1989) Family food systems, preventive health and dietary change: a policy to increase the health divide. *Journal of Social Policy* **18**(2), 167–85.

World Health Organization Regional Office for Europe and The Centre for Public Health Research (1994) *Training and Research in Public Health: Policy Perspectives for a 'New Public Health'* Training and Research in Public Health Dialogue Series No.1, Karlstad 15/2/95.

CHAPTER 12

Research to support health promotion based on community development approaches

Frances Baum

INTRODUCTION

This chapter explores the ways in which research can support health promotion that uses a community development approach. To do this it is necessary to describe briefly the ways in which health promotion has changed over the past two decades, from a focus on disease and its prevention in individuals to a focus on health and the structures that promote or detract from it. Not surprisingly, the broadening of the approaches used in health promotion has challenged researchers to be more creative and eclectic in inventing ways in which research can support those engaged in developing new ways of promoting health (Colquhoun and Kellehear, 1993).

What are the characteristics of the new approaches to health promotion? Health promotion has been re-evaluated in the past decade. Until the early 1980s the dominant paradigm focused on individuals, exhorting them to change their behaviour and lifestyle in ways that would be more likely to leave them healthy. Thus people were encouraged to take more exercise, eat a diet low in fat and high in fibre, with fresh fruit and vegetables, and conduct routine self-examination for various cancers. While these approaches may certainly have contributed to health, the 1980s saw an increasing recognition that factors affecting health are more complex than simply peoples' behaviours, and that some people are better positioned to change their behaviour than others.

Individuals' income level, educational level, employment status, genetic inheritance, quality of housing, working environment, neighbourhood social environment, and the quality of the physical environment all interact in determining the available options, and eventually their health status. This recognition led health promoters in the mid-1980s to devise strategies that attempted to tackle the broad range of factors that make up the matrix of influences on health. The most prominent of these has been the World Health Organization's Healthy Cities project (Kickbusch, 1989; Tsouros, 1990; Ashton, 1992). Healthy Cities sees health promotion as primarily an issue for communities as a whole working together rather than as activities focusing on individuals (Dulh and Hancock, 1988; Evers *et al.*, 1990). The premises of the approach are that:

- health is a social rather than a medical matter;
- health is the responsibility of all city services;
- health is an outcome of collaborative action between community members, planners and providers of public and private services;
- health should be monitored by physical, social, aesthetic and environmental indicators of wellbeing;
- a city or community should promote health in an active way.

Since the original European project was established in 1986, the idea of Healthy Cities has spread rapidly. By 1990 it was claimed to be a movement rather than just a project (Tsouros, 1990), and projects have been started across the world, endorsed by the World Health Organization. Australia had a pilot project in three cities (Canberra; Noarlunga, South Australia; Wollongong, New South Wales). Alongside the officially labelled Healthy Cities projects, many other cities and communities across the world have been experimenting with health promotion initiatives that aim to tackle the underlying and structural causes of illness and disease. Some of these have been based in local community or womens' community health centres, others in local government or local community groups. Very often the initiatives involve a combination of local groups and organizations working togther with the common aim of promoting health locally.

Typically these projects, whether they are labelled Healthy Cities or not, will use the techniques of community development. Perhaps the most significant feature of community development work is that it involves a partnership between people in a particular locality working alongside paid professionals to identify concerns and then devise and implement strategies to address the concerns. Butler and Cass (1993a) provide documentation of health promotion based on community development techniques. This approach is quite different from health promotion work in a community, which is based on issues identified by health or other professionals rather than by local people. Such projects appear not to tackle complex social and environmental problems, such as the powerlessness of people living on low incomes, the development of social networks or problems of local environmental pollution. Work around the world suggests that when local communities are consulted about health issues of concern to them, they invariably see those to do with their living, working and environmental conditions as the ones of most importance.

Examples of community development health promotion include a number of the initiatives under the Noarlunga Healthy Cities programme. These worked on pollution of the local river, advocacy for improved public transport and defence of a local community from stigmatizing by the press (see Baum *et al.*, 1992 for details). Butler and Cass (1993b) provide a series of case studies of community development. These include descriptions of the development of a community food cooperative, bushfire education and residents' action groups.

HOW RESEARCH CAN SUPPORT NEW APPROACHES TO HEALTH PROMOTION

Healthy Cities and other community health promotion initiatives are usually challenging established practice and advocating new ways of doing things. Consequently, research to support the planning, implementation and evaluation of the approaches can be very useful in what may often not be an entirely supportive environment. Research can serve to legitimize and validate activities that might not otherwise be taken seriously by power brokers. Most projects of the Healthy Cities type have a natural history that will involve planning, implementation and evaluation. Research can assist the initiative's development at each of these stages. The research involved is, as this chapter will reveal, very applied and should be directly applicable to the organizational and community concerns. This chapter will describe the ways in which research can assist in each stage of these health promotion projects, and then go on to discuss some general methodological guidelines.

Deciding what to do: needs assessment and planning

The social understanding of health, on which the new approaches to health promotion are built, provides a seemingly endless list of issues that could be tackled by health promoters: there is no area of life that is not of potential concern to them. Community needs assessments are often seen as the starting point for deciding what priorities should be pursued (see South Australian Community Health Research Unit, 1991, for a detailed guide to conducting community health needs assessments). Many of these have been conducted in local communities in recent years. Usually they involve the collation of data from bodies such as the Australian Bureau of Statistics about the community in question. The types of data collected are shown in Table 12.1. Often quantitative data are collected by surveying a community sample, and possibly some qualitative data are collected from local residents. These are then used to determine the priorities for action of the health promoting group or organization.

Table 12.1 Checklist of information likely to be useful for planning healthy communities

Topics	Type of information
People	
Demography population make-up and epidemiology of illness	Total population, age distribution, birth and fertility rate, death rates, house-hold types, income and employment profiles, ethnic profile, languages spoken. Main causes of morbidity and mortality.
Perceptions of area	Residents' views about desirability, safety, nature of area. Attitudes and beliefs concerning health and illness and available services. Perceptions of key health problems. Perceptions of strengths of community.
Support networks	Contact between residents, informal caring, methods of information dispersal, social interaction, community 'hub(s)' (or lack of); what is the impetus or driving force of this interaction?
Community norms, values and traditions, history	A feel for local beliefs and variations in these. Awareness of local ethnic groups; their attitudes, values, concerns. Presence or absence of significant museums, festivals, traditional rituals. Religious expressions and involvement in health-related concerns. Gender-relations; their expression in domestic and wider social life. Print and electronic media; state and local.
Locality and infrastructure	
Housing and planning	Overview of type and suitability of housing. Adequacy of planning and provision of services. Housing needs of different groups (e.g. young people and those with disabilities). Private and public ownership; rental market.

Topics	Type of Information
Transport	Level of vehicle ownership. Adequacy of public transport provision for bicycle tracks – perceived gaps.
Water, sewerage, energy sources	Availability and type of supply. Note inadequacy.
Organizations and services	
State and local government	Inventory of local services (with focus on health and welfare), and professional and non-professional perceptions of gaps. Extent of cooperation or conflict between agencies.
Non-government and community groups	Inventory of these, including self-help groups, and lobbying groups. Actual and potential involvement in health promotion.
Intersectoral groups	Social planning committees, community forums.
Business and economic	Main businesses and trades (including business in the home). Occupational health provision, unions. Occupational illnesses and accidents.
Administration and power	Analysis of administrative structure and politics (federal, state and local government; lobby groups). Perceptions of power holders and others. Analysis of extent of communication between different sectors and levels of government. Assessment of ability of the community to influence decision-making. Where is power centred? Balance/imbalance of health-related expenditure. Clinical/medical health vs. social/community health.
Natural environment	
Climate, geography, environmental health	Description of location, rainfall, temperature ranges, topography, etc. Air and water quality/pollution.

This process sounds like a fairly straightforward research exercise, but in practice it is rarely as uncomplicated as it sounds. The following issues pose particular problems in conducting needs assessment.

Timing

Conducting needs assessment research of the type described above does not happen very quickly. Surveys take time to plan (especially when a number of agencies and organizations are involved), pilot, conduct and analyse. Agencies often commence a needs assessment and find that they do not have the resources to complete it, or that they have to make crucial decisions before the information is available. An important issue, then, is for those involved in needs assessment to tailor the exercise to the particular purpose. It is little use having data when the opportunity to use it has passed. Although organizations may only conduct a substantial needs assessment occasionally, they need to develop way of listening to their local community and receiving feedback on its changing needs and priorities on an ongoing basis.

Skills

Needs assessments are often conducted by health workers, who have often not had training in survey and qualitative research methods. They are usually trained with a heavy focus on the skills needed for individual treatment rather than on those for a population approach to health promotion. Without some knowledge or a good source of advice needs assessment can go badly wrong. Such an instance came to my attention recently. A rural health service had attempted a survey of all residents in their area. They achieved only an 8% response rate, added to which was the fact that the questionnaire was poorly designed, which meant that the survey exercise yielded very little useful information.

Values

Like most research, needs assessment reflects the values of those conducting it. It is not uncommon to find those doing the assessment expressing the hope that they will be able to collect 'scientific data that will be value-free'. In practice, community health needs assessments are deeply imbued with values. Those setting out with a medical model of health will collect quite different data from those operating within a social perspective (Baum, 1988). The interpretations put on the data are also likely to differ. The former approach would concentrate on information about illness and disease and use of health services. The latter would also encompass information about living conditions, employment, housing and perceptions of the environment. A key concern of a social perspective on health would be a focus on equity in health status and how this could be worked towards at a local level. In health, the interpretation of reasons for inequities in status demonstrates how crucial values and world views are to making sense of data. This is well demonstrated in Townsend and

Davidson's (1982) book on inequalities in health in Britain. The authors put forward four main categories of explanation: that the inequalities were simply an artefact of the measurement technique; that they reflected natural or social selection; that they reflected the structural and material conditions of peoples' lives; or that they reflected behavioural and cultural mores by which people chose to live their lives. Subsequent authors have offered further interpretations of the data (Powles and Salzberg, 1989). Theoretical and value differences are just as crucial in local, seemingly atheoretical, empirical research. Needs assessment reports should discuss such issues of interpretation and make transparent the values of the researchers. Some such research conducted in South Australia has done this (Baum and Abbott, 1989). A report on correlations between income and reported health status was discussed in terms of alternative interpretation of the data. The researchers stated their view that this difference was due to the life circumstances of individuals, but they noted that this contrasted with the views of people they had consulted who saw low-income people's less advantageous health status as resulting from their reckless behaviour and failure to look after their own health.

Lateral and creative thinking

Needs assessment exercises should be carried out in such a way that the process encourages those involved to be thoughtful and reflective. Ideally it should encourage them to think laterally and challenge the current practice and mode of operation of their organization. It has been noted that health professionals have a tendency to discover a 'need' for the services they offer. Thus in relation to the problem of widespread prevalence of back pain a chiropractor may see the need for more chiropractic services, an orthopaedic specialist for more provision for their specialty in a hospital budget, a physiotherapist for more of their service and an ergonomist for more ergonomic assessment in workplaces. Short (1989) describes an incidence in the Illawarra (NSW) community in which professional interests, in her view, 'manipulated' community opinion to see a need for a linear accelerator for cancer treatment, at a cost of $1.5 million. She argues that alternative uses of the money, such as health promotion, environmental clean-up or palliative care, were not considered in the public debate. This case illustrates the political nature of the definition of need. A researcher external to those with a strong commitment could be powerful in challenging taken-for-granted professional agendas, and encouraging workers and others to take a broader view of a particular issue. This is particularly important in relation to health promotion, when those trained in the health sciences so easily opt for solutions aimed at individuals rather than considering the range of possible interventions available to promote health. Arguing for health promotion as a need, especially community-driven health promotion, is likely to be difficult in a climate of scarce resources and media promotion of the 'miracles' of curative medicine. Well formulated research can play a role in informing and challenging the debate on health resource allocation.

Ensuring the difference between a problem and a solution is well defined

Needs assessments are sometimes characterized by a tendency for those involved in them to jump straight to defining a solution before fully analysing a particular issue or problem. Needs research should build in mechanisms that protect the assessment from this tendency. An example might be that a solution to a defined need might be stated as 'Socially isolated older people in our community need a volunteer visitors scheme'. The problem is that the research has found that there are a significant proportion of people in the community who are lonely because they do not have places to go and do not have private transport. Alternative solutions would be provide community transport to enable these people to move around the community, to organize group activities or to encourage people to make friends in their own neighbourhood. The need assessment process should encourage those involved in the needs assessment and the organization(s) whose activities it is designed to shape to apply analysis and thought to the data they collect and not to expect the data to 'speak for themselves'.

Part of the trick of teasing out problems from solutions lies in providing communities with relevant and accessible information that will encourage community debate, involvement and, hopefully, resolution of a health issue. Such information can be crucial to building a critical momentum for change.

The process of data collection should be recognized as the starting point for the organization or project to plan their work. A recent report on strategic planning in community health (Sanderson, 1993) argues that the process is more akin to sailing than driving along a road. Like sailing, strategic planning has to take into account multiple factors that have an impact on the decisions taken. These will include local political circumstances, skills of available resource people, philosophies of funding bodies, local information collected in the needs assessment and the topics for which those involved feel some passion.

EVALUATION

There has been an increasing focus on the evaluation of human services in general, and of health services in particular. Health workers and others are called upon to demonstrate the 'health gain', the outcome and the direct benefits of the interventions they have planned. There is a plethora of literature relating to evaluation. Because of space constraints this section will not provide a how-to-do-it guide: there are many of these available (Hawe *et al.*, 1990; Wadsworth, 1991; SACHRU, 1994a). General methodological issues are, however, taken up in the following section. Here I will concentrate on the political and organizational issues. These projects are particularly challenging to evaluators because they typically have developing objectives that change over the course of the exercise, directly reflect their social and political context, and aim to bring about change in rather vague and difficult to define concepts such as empowerment and social connectedness.

Around Australia health services are being subjected to reorganizations which have the supposed aim of improving efficiency and effectiveness. Much emphasis is placed on assessing costs and putting precise monetary values on particular interventions. The main evaluative outcome appears to be value for money (Petersen, 1994). In this context community-based health promotion faces a particularly difficult challenge. It is hard enough for treatment services to demonstrate any direct impact on individuals in terms of health status. Local community work is generally low-budget, long-term, and has a focus on processes and developing competencies rather than direct health outcomes (Baum and Cooke, 1992; Baum, 1993). It is not easy to evaluate in terms of cost-effectiveness. Increasingly, however, community health services are under pressure to do just this. These unrealistic pressures tend to make community health managers and workers less amenable to the concept of evaluation.

Conducting evaluations is never easy. Service providers are busy people who usually have more demands on their time than they have time available, and so evaluation is rarely a top priority. It may also threaten people and organizations. Most health workers and managers are familiar with the rhetoric which says that they should include evaluation as part of their routine work, but in practice it is rare that this happens. The mid-1990s are witnessing considerable cutbacks in public expenditure on health services, and the pressures this imposes on agencies often means that evaluation takes even more of a back seat. Researchers conducting or wanting to conduct evaluations in partnership with agencies have to be aware of the context of the organization and people they hope to work with. Negotiating entry to an agency is a crucial stage in any evaluation. This is obviously far easier if you are invited by the organization to conduct the evaluation. The motivation to cooperate is then established. Even so, not everyone involved in the intervention will be equally willing to cooperate. If you are not invited then the task of negotiating the evaluation is more challenging. You may be a student who wants to do an evaluation as part of your studies, and as such you may or may not be an employee of the organization. In primary health care and public health an increasing number of workers are studying postgraduate courses while in paid employment. They are likely to be keen to do their research in an area related to their work, and evaluation is very often a candidate for this. Being clear about the basis on which the evaluation is being conducted and whether the preconditions for successful evaluation are in place is crucial. Researchers and managers need to agree on the following questions.

Is the initiative ready to be evaluated?

This means ensuring that it is not too early to conduct an evaluation and that it could reasonably be expected that the initiative has had an opportunity to have an impact.

Do the key people associated with the intervention (including professional and community people involved) want it to be evaluated? Are they keen to cooperate? If the answer to these questions is no, then it will be difficult to conduct an evaluation. Cooperation from key players is very important. There are many ways in which an evaluation exercise can be subverted.

What are the politics associated with the evaluation?

Evaluation is inevitably a political process. Whoever conducts an evaluation cannot avoid being tied up with organizational politics, and possibly broader political agendas. Inevitably, community development in health projects involves a range of vested interests (Hunt, 1987; Marsden and Oakley, 1991; Baum and Cooke, 1992). Professionals, funding bodies and community people will all have different perspectives and expectations of any particular intervention. An evaluator should attempt to assess the politics of the setting of their evaluation and will have to keep a constant watch for the impact of political issues as the evaluation proceeds. A good evaluation incorporates the complexities of any situation (Furler, 1979) but does not become so complex that its findings are too dense to be useful (Wadsworth, 1991).

Are there sufficient resources to conduct the evaluation?

Evaluation costs money. The scope and approach of any evaluation has to be tailored to the available resources. As a rough rule of thumb a community health promotion project should consider spending approximately 10% of the cost of an intervention on evaluation. If managers and funders expect evaluation to be done then resources have to be provided. If the evaluation design requires the project staff to collect information then the researcher must ensure they have the time to do this and are willing to do so. If the evaluation is being conducted by project staff then they must ensure that they set aside sufficient time to conduct and write it up. Community workers are often very action-orientated and may be reluctant to spend time on documenting and producing reports. This is where a researcher working in partnership can be of great assistance. They can become the voice of a project and its achievements and challenges, and ensure that these are documented so that they can contribute to broader debates.

Are the necessary skills available?

Ideally all health promotion and community development staff would have well-developed skills in evaluation. Sometimes this is the case, but more commonly such skills are not strong or seen as a priority. A recent review of a national health promotion funding programme in South Australia (SACHRU, 1994b) reported that many of the officers employed on the funded projects felt that they did not have well-developed evaluation skills. This had made evaluating their projects difficult, even though some formal evaluation advice had been organized for them.

How will feedback on the evaluation be given?

Giving feedback is an important aspect of evaluation research and is crucial to ensuring that the findings from an evaluation get used. It is helpful if methods for doing this can be negotiated in advance. If the feedback happens in such a way that those receiving it reject it, then no action is likely to result. Ideally, in an evaluation process there should be enough interaction to ensure that the key findings come as no surprise to any of the main parties involved. Possibly the sign of a good evaluation is when people comment: 'I could have told you that'. Although this is not very rewarding for the evaluator, it is one indicator that they have conducted their evaluation effectively (Patton *et al.*, 1977).

Who should conduct the evaluation?

Evaluation can be conducted by the people responsible for the particular programme – an insider's evaluation. Alternatively it may be conducted by outsiders. There are advantages and some drawbacks to both approaches. Table 12.2 summarizes these (Feuerstein, 1986).

There is no inherent benefit to either approach. The decision on which to choose will depend on the resources available, the purpose of doing the evaluation, the requirements of funding bodies, and the stage of the intervention being evaluated. The important thing is that the choice should be thought through as part of the planning stage.

SHAPING METHODOLOGIES FOR HEALTH PROMOTION BASED ON COMMUNITY DEVELOPMENT

The following guidelines are designed to be applicable to research used in community health promotion regardless of its purpose. They are generally points that are relevant to each of the categories of activities mentioned above.

Table 12.2 The advantages and disadvantages of external and internal evaluators

External	Internal
Can take a 'fresh' look at the programme.	Knows the programme only too well.
Not personally involved, so it is easier to be objective.	Finds it hardest to be objective.
Is not a part of the normal power structure.	Is a part of the power and authority structure.
Gains nothing from the programme, but may gain prestige from the evaluation.	May be motivated by hopes of personal gain.
Trained in evaluation methods. May have experience in other evaluations. Regarded as an 'expert' by the programme.	May not be specially trained in evaluation methods. Has no more (or only a little more) training than others in the programme.
An 'outsider' who may not understand the programme or the people involved.	Is familiar with and understands the programme, and can interpret personal behaviour and attitudes.
May cause anxiety as programme staff and participants are not sure of his or her motives.	Known to the programme, so poses no threat of anxiety or disruption. Final recommendations may appear less threatening.

Reproduced with permission (from Feuerstein, 1986, p.10)

Participation in Research

Partners in research

Participation by practitioners and communities in research relevant to them is being recognized as the hallmark of good practice. Traditionally, research has been conducted in universities by students and academics in isolation from other interests. This position is changing, and governments and organizations and community groups conduct their own research, or employ consultants to do so. University-based researchers are under increasing pressure to make and maintain strong links with practitioners in public health as much as any other field. O'Neill (1993) describes an attempt in Canada to bring together health promotion practitioners and academics from a range of disciplines. He reported the exercise as highlighting rather than breaking down the barriers to multidisciplinary cooperation.

This Knowledge Development project invited academics to play a role different from their usual one of 'defining and dominating knowledge development'. Rather, the project asked them to give away some of this power and work in partnership with practitioners in such a way that their knowledge, drawn from practice, was respected. The project used the term 'knowledge' rather than 'research' to place the focus on the range of knowledge that is developed in service agencies and grassroots organizations. O'Neill (1993) reports that building bridges between the practical and academic world is not easy. He concludes that one of the crucial aspects of a successful recipe is continuity of effort and funding. This will ensure that networks and alliances can be fuelled by trust that develops over time. This experience certainly echoes the South Australian experience, where a community health research unit has been funded by the state health department over 10 years, and this has enabled effective links to be developed by the researchers and community health centres. Maintaining academic credibility (essential to obtaining grants) and strong links with a university health faculty, convincing a health department of the value of continuing to fund research and being an activist in a marginalized community health movement is a tricky balancing exercise, as the author can testify. These juggling skills appear likely to be important for researchers in the coming years, as research is increasingly valued for its practical application.

Benefits for communities and researchers

Since Health for All, there has been an increasing recognition of the potential for community participation in the planning, implementation and evaluation of health programmes. The Healthy Cities movement has reinforced this. Such participation is at the heart of attempts to promote health using a community development framework. The emphasis on participation in part reflects a disenchantment with reliance on experts for knowledge about particular issues. A further recognition is that professionals can become as concerned about advancing the cause of their profession as they are about the people their profession is designed to serve (Freidson, 1970; Willis, 1983). It also comes from a recognition that local people are often experts on their own needs and those of their communities. Public health researchers often fail to consult professional workers, let alone communities. However, it is now being recognized that good public health research generally results from involving the key groups affected by a particular piece of research. The Healthy Cities network, which links researchers around the world, has consistently emphasized this aspect of research practice (de Leeuw *et al.*, 1993; Davies and Kelly, 1993; Baum and Brown, 1989).

Much has been written and said about the benefits of participation: actual examples of research that is consultative or participatory are rarer.

Most research that is sensitive to the need to involve communities is consultative rather than participatory. In community development research it is crucial to ensure that the research is integrated with the initiative and built in in the early stages of planning. Advisory committees can be a useful way of involving a broad range of people. While it takes time and effort to encourage people to give up their time to be on such a committee, and although using the committee may slow down the progress of the project, the benefits in terms of grounding the project in the concerns of health professionals and community members are real. In the case of needs assessment the committee can be a valuable source of information, as well as helping to ensure that the output from the research is used in the local area.

There is a reduced tolerance of research practices that are not consultative. Professionals and community members alike express scepticism at vague statements about the likely benefits of research. Unless people believe in the value of the research they are unlikely to participate. They are more likely to do so if the research is clearly of benefit to them or their community. Such scepticism is entirely reasonable. Wadsworth (1984) has dubbed much research a 'data raid', in which researchers swoop down from their ivory tower, collect data, whisk back to their tower and never communicate their findings to the people who were their subjects. Professional workers may also be cynical about research. They know evaluations are often conducted for reasons other than a genuine attempt to review initiative, and that the findings are often distorted by political processes. If, however, they have a sense of control over and involvement in a project, they are much more likely to be committed both to the research process and to taking action on the basis of its findings. The commitment of professionals to research is only likely to happen in a busy – and usually overstretched – service delivery agency if managers are supportive of the research effort and give it legitimacy, and therefore credibility. Researchers should therefore seek to establish good working relationships with the managers of services they aim to work with. With a few exceptions (Feuerstein, 1986; Marsden and Oakley, 1991; Wadsworth, 1991), textbooks on research methods do not pay much attention to the involvement in the process of people other than researchers. Other participants tend to be seen as passive.

Community-driven research

Research may be conducted by community groups in a direct attempt to influence policy and practice related to their community health. In South Australia residents in the northwest suburbs of Adelaide conducted their own survey of residents' perceptions of air pollution. Their report, *If You Don't Like it Move*, proved to be an effective instrument for lobbying government and local industries. While there were attempts to discredit the report's methodology, the concerns expressed by residents received some recognition from government and industry. There is now a local environmental forum, with local and state government officials, health workers, residents and industry represented. The survey was one of a range of lobbying and activist strategies used by the local action group. Such use of research by local groups on issues of public health importance is an effective way of influencing policy and local public health (Wadsworth, 1988).

METHODOLOGICAL ECLECTICISM

Research to support health promotion in the community should be methodologically eclectic, selecting those methods that are most likely to illuminate issues rather than being committed to any particular methodology. Many authors have argued this view (Furler, 1979; Brown, 1975; Owen and Mohr, 1986; Baum and Brown, 1989; Scott-Samuel, 1989; Daly and Willis, 1990; Patton, 1990; Baum, 1994).

Data should also be interpreted in the light of relevant theories. In both needs assessment and evaluation research a range of methodologies can be utilized to assist understanding and develop knowledge. In particular, the value of qualitative methodologies has been recognized in recent years (Daly and Willis, 1990; Miller and Crabtree, 1992; Holman, 1993). These are particularly appropriate for discovering the meaning of social practices, the importance of a particular social context and an understanding of actions taken by individuals. Such understanding is important to determining need and assessing the impact of a development initiative on the health of a community.

This book is testimony to the fact that in any areas of health the plurality of methods used is increasing. Many methods used come from the social sciences. They are not new: most have a long and respectable history. They are, however, often new to public health, which has tended to draw on medicine and its scientific premises rather than on the many bodies of knowledge and methodologies within social science. In fact, there probably is not a discipline within social science that does not have a significant contribution to make to our knowledge and understanding of the new public health. For example, a political scientist's analysis of power relations within cities could prove to be an invaluable tool for an evaluator of a Healthy Cities project who is trying to make sense of why certain actors dominated the project, or why the rhetoric of participation proved so hard to implement. An understanding of decision-making theory and organizational culture would be important for an evaluation of a community development campaign that aimed to change the practice of a local industry perceived as a source of pollution by local residents. Despite this potential, theories that abound in each social science discipline are rarely used as effectively as they might be by health promotion researchers. But the need to extend the methodological and theoretical net used by public health researchers is now being recognized (see, for example, the Leeds Declaration (WHO and Yorkshire Health, 1993; Bunton and Macdonald, 1992). At the heart of good research practice for health promotion should be a strong emphasis on critical appraisal. It is through this that those involved in the research process are able to enhance the validity of their data and the conclusions drawn from them. Such appraisal implies a willingness to draw conclusions that challenge accepted practice. Given that most community develoment approaches to health are deeply embedded in local circumstances, research should reflect an undersanding of the impact of this complex setting on local needs identification or the evaluation of, for example, the achievements of a local advocacy group. Successful research in this context is likely to be methodologically pluralistic, reflect critical, creative and lateral thought, and be grounded in a sound understanding of social and political theory and of the processes by which social change occurs.

ENSURING THAT RESEARCH RESULTS ARE USED

Researchers should ensure that evaluation and needs assessment research are used. Cynicism about research is increased when people see that it makes no difference to practice. In the case of needs assessment a well-prepared report or set of reports should be able to influence planning for a number of years, and enable health promotion practitioners to shift towards an approach to health promotion which conforms to the criteria outlined in the introduction. As explained in the evaluation section, evaluation results should be discussed and assessed by key players as soon as is practicable. Much community health promotion goes unreported and so remains invisible. It is important that experiences are shared between communities so that a body of knowledge and theory about the practice of health promotion and community development is constructed. Because these initiatives are challenging to evaluate and often operate on a shoestring, this has not yet happened to any extent. The type of broader questions raised by these approaches to health promotion include:

- How can government agencies best operate to increase the opportunities for community input into their planning and evaluation?
- Is the community involvement real or rhetorical?
- Under what conditions can community development health promotion bring about significant change to promote health?
- Is community development more about social control than change that promotes social justice?
- What factors make for effective cooperation between different sectors (including the community) in efforts to improve health in local communities?

These questions deserve more exploration if health promoters are to come to grips with the challenge of promoting health in communities that have fewer resources and skills than others.

Such theory building is of most interest to academics and practitioners. Community members are more likely to want to know how the information relates to their particular situation, whether it be as a member of an action group, user of a service, member of a Board of Management, local government councillor or a citizen concerned about local health issues. These people have a right to expect researchers to produce reports that are readily accessible to them. Guidelines for such reports indicate that they should:

- be simply written and as free of jargon as possible;
- be illustrated with pictures and/or cartoons or other graphics;
- present numerical data in an attractive way so that it is accessible to people without highly developed statistical skills;
- be attractive to look at and concise.

Fortunately, the availability of increasingly easy to use desktop publishing systems makes this feasible. Research can also be reported in more creative ways through the use of video, strip cartoons and community art. Launching reports such as a community needs assessment with a local dignitary can be an important part of the publicity process, maximizing the chance that research findings will be utilized. Obviously media skills are useful here.

CONCLUSION

New approaches to health promotion offer exciting opportunities for researchers who are keen to utilize their practical skills as part of a process of social change and development. Community activities are not easy to plan, evaluate and theorize about. The complexities of the natural history of these projects means that researchers have to be inventive with the techniques they use, communicate effectively to develop partnerships with community practitioners and the communities they work with, and manage to keep their theoretical heads above the day-to-day hubbub of community action to see how the particular case fits more general knowledge and theory. This research will never be as confined and manageable as that involved with health promotion concerned with more defined variables (such as weight loss or smoking cessation), but it does hold great promise for contributing to signifcant changes in the health of local communities.

AUTHOR'S NOTE

The author wishes to thank Paul Laris and Libby Kalucy for commenting on a final draft of this chapter.

REFERENCES

Ashton, J. (1992) *Healthy Cities*, Open University Press, Milton Keynes.

Baum, F. (1988) Community-based research for promoting the new public health. *Health Promotion* 3(3), 259–67.

Baum, F. (1993) Noarlunga Healthy Cities Pilot Project – the contribution of research and evaluation, in *Healthy Cities Research and Practice*, eds J.K. Davies and M. Kelly, Routledge, London, pp. 90–111.

Baum, F. (1994) Researching public health: behind the qualitative–quantitative methodological debate. *Social Science and Medicine* (in press).

Baum, F. and Abbott, D. (1989) *A Social Health Perspective*. A report from the Marion, Brighton and Glenelg Community Health needs assessment, Adelaide: South Australian Community Health Research Unit.

Baum, F. and Brown, V. (1989) Healthy Cities (Australia) Project: issues of evaluation for the new public health. *Community Health Studies* 13(2), 140–9.

Baum, F. and Cooke, R. (1992) Healthy Cities Australia: The evaluation of the pilot project in Noarlunga, South Australia. *Health Promotion International* 7(3), 181–93.

Baum, F., Traynor, M. and Brice, G. (1992) Healthy Cities: the Noarlunga experience, in *Health Policy Development, Implementation and Evaluation in Australia*, ed H. Gardner, Churchill Livingstone, Melbourne, Chapter 14.

Brown, V. (1985) Towards an epidemiology of health: a basis for planning community health programs. *Health Policy* 4, 331–40.

Bunton, R. and Macdonald, G. (eds) (1992) *Health Promotion – Disciplines and Diversity*, Routledge, London.

Butler, P. and Cass, S. (eds) (1993a) *Community Health Studies* 13. Proceedings from Australian Community Health Association Conference.

Butler, P. and Cass, S. (eds) (1993b) *Case Studies of Community Development in Health*, Centre for Development and Innovation in Health, Melbourne.

Colquhoun, D. and Kellehear, A. (eds) (1993) *Health Research in Practice: Political, Ethical and Methodological Issues*, Chapman & Hall, London.

Daly, J. and Willis E. (eds) (1990) *Social Sciences and Health Research*, Public Health Association of Australia, Canberra.

Davies, J.K. and Kelly, M. (eds) (1993) *Healthy Cities Research and Practice*, Routledge, London.

de Leeuw, E., O'Neill, M., Goumans, M. and de Bruijn, F. (eds) (1993) *Healthy Cities Research Agenda*. Proceedings of an expert panel, Maastricht, The Netherlands: Research for Health Cities Clearing House, University of Limburg.

Dulh, L. and Hancock, T. (1988) *A Guide to Assessing Healthy Cities*, WHO Healthy Cities Papers No. 3, FADL Publishers, Copenhagen.

Evers, A., Farrant, W. and Trojan, A. (eds) (1990) *Healthy Public Policy at a Local Level*, Canpus Verlag, Frankfurt.

Feuerstein, M.-T. (1986) *Partners in Evaluation*, Macmillan, London.

Freidson, E. (1970) *Professional Dominance: The Social Structure of Medical Care*, Aldine, Chicago.

Furler, E. (1979) Against hegemony in health care service evaluation. *Community Health Studies* 3(1), 32–41.

Hawe, P., Degeling, D. and Hall, J. (1990) *Evaluating Health Promotion: A Health Workers's Guide*, MacLennan and Petty, Sydney.

Holman, H.R. (1993) Qualitative inquiry in medical research. *Journal of Clinical Epidemiology* 46, 29–36.

Hunt, S.M. (1987) Evaluating a community development project – issues of acceptability. *British Journal of Social Work* 17, 661–7.

Kickbusch, I. (1989) *Good Planets are Hard to Find*. WHO Healthy Cities papers No. 5, Copenhagen: European Regional Office of the World Health Organization.

Marsden, D. and Oakley, P. (1991) Future issues and perspectives in the evaluation of social development, *Community Development Journal* 26(4), 315–28.

Miller, W.L. and Crabtree, B.F. (1992) Primary care research: a multi-method typology and qualitative road map, in *Doing Qualitative Research*, eds B.F. Crabtree and W.L. Miller, Sage Publications, Newbury Park, California, Chapter 1.

O'Neill, M. (1993) Building bridges between knowledge and action: the Canadian process of Healthy Communities indicators, in *Healthy Cities Research and Practice*, eds J.K. Davies and M. Kelly, Routledge, London, Chapter 10.

Owen, A. and Mohr, R. (1986) Politics and pitfalls in evaluation. *Community Health Studies* 10(1), 95–9.

Patton, M.Q. (1990) *Qualitative Evaluation and Research Methods*, Sage Publications, Newbury Park, California.

Patton, M.Q., Grimes, P.S., Gutherie, K.M. *et al.* (1977) In search of impact: an analysis of the utilization of federal health evaluation research, in *Using Social Research in Public Policy Making*, ed C.H. Weiss, Lexington Books, New York.

Petersen, A.R. (1994) Bureaucracies, rational experts and health, in *In a Critical Condition – Health and Power Relations in Australia*, Allen and Unwin, Sydney, Chapter 5.

Powles, J. and Salzberg, M.(1989) Work, class or lifestyle? Explaining inequalities in health, in *Sociology of Health and Illness: Australian Readings*, eds G. Lupton and J.M. Najman, MacMillan, Melbourne, Chapter 7, pp. 135–168.

Sanderson, C. (1993) *From Strategic Planning to Strategic Thinking, Results of a Study on the Practice of Strategic Planning in South Australian Community Health Centres*, SACHRU, Adelaide.

Scott-Samuel, A.(1989) Building the new public health: a public health alliance and a new social epidemiology, in *Readings for a New Public Health*, eds C. Martin and D.V. McQueen, Edinburgh University Press, Edinburgh, pp. 29–41.

Short, S. (1989) Community participation or community manipulation? A case study of the Illawarra cancer appeal-a-thon. *Community Health Studies* 13(1), 34–8.

South Australian Community Health Research Unit (1991) *Planning Healthy Communities*, SACHRU, Adelaide.

South Australian Community Health Research Unit (1994a) *How to Evaluate Your Community Health Programs*, Paper No. 2 in Research and Evaluation in Community Health Series, SACHRU, Adelaide.

South Australian Community Health Research Unit (1994b) *Evaluation of the South Australian Component of the National Better Health Program*, SACHRU, Adelaide.

Townsend, P. and Davidson, N. (1982) *Inequalities in Health: the Black Report*, Penguin, Harmondsworth.

Tsouros, A. (1990) *World Health Organization Healthy Cities Project: A Project Becomes a Movement*, FADL Publishers, Copenhagen.

Wadsworth, Y. (1984) *Do-It-Yourself Social Research*, Victorian Council of Social Services, Melbourne.

Wadsworth, Y. (1988) *Participatory Research and Development in Primary Health Care by Community Groups*, Report to the NHMRC, Public Health Research and Development Committee, Consumers Health Forum, Canberra.

Wadsworth, Y. (1991) *Everyday Evaluation On the Run*, Action Research Issues Association (Inc.), Melbourne.

Willis, E. (1983) *Medical Dominance*, George Allen and Unwin, Sydney.

World Health Organization and Yorkshire Health (1993) *The Leeds Declaration – Principles for Action*, Nuffield Institute for Health, University of Leeds, Leeds.

Index